PRAISE FOR *PLANTIFULLY SIMPLE*

"Plantifully Simple is a must-read for anyone looking to optim[...] [well]-being. Whether you are fully plant-based or just want to improve nutrition for a nourished body and mind, Kiki's recipes and guidance are sure to set you up for success! She writes in a wonderfully warm and inviting way, and this is carried through her healthy and delicious recipes."

—Dr. Uma Naidoo, author of *This Is Your Brain on Food* and *Calm Your Mind with Food*

"The weight-loss industry is full of misleading, confusing, and factually incorrect information. In Kiki's new masterpiece, you'll finally have the blueprint to sustainable weight loss. Why is it sustainable? Because the meals are simple, science backed, and wildly delicious!"

—Robby Barbaro, MPH, coauthor of *Mastering Diabetes*

"Plantifully Simple is nothing short of a breath of fresh air in the world of tired weight-loss regimens and diet cults. . . . Kiki's deep understanding of nutritional science makes this book a must-have for anyone who's serious about their health and well-being. . . . Prepare to be inspired and delighted with every recipe you try."

—Matt Tullman, cofounder and CEO of No Meat Athlete

"Kiki Nelson knows how to reinvent herself, her mindset, and her meal plans to achieve and maintain weight loss with a healthy, plant-based diet. In *Plantifully Simple*, she shows us precisely how we can do it, too. With delicious, nourishing recipes, her program is designed to work for the long haul. It's time to stop dieting and start embracing a proven lifestyle approach to a better and healthier you."   **—Robert Cheeke, *New York Times* bestselling coauthor of *The Plant-Based Athlete***

Plantifully
Simple

Plantifully
Simple

100 Plant-Based Recipes and Meal Plans for Health and Weight Loss

KIKI NELSON

WITH RACHEL HOLTZMAN

SIMON ELEMENT

NEW YORK LONDON TORONTO SYDNEY NEW DELHI

SIMON
ELEMENT

An Imprint of Simon & Schuster, LLC
1230 Avenue of the Americas
New York, NY 10020

First Simon Element hardcover edition July 2024

SIMON ELEMENT is a trademark of Simon & Schuster, LLC

Simon & Schuster: Celebrating 100 Years of Publishing in 2024

For information about special discounts for bulk purchases, please contact Simon & Schuster Special Sales at 1-866-506-1949 or business@simonandschuster.com.

The Simon & Schuster Speakers Bureau can bring authors to your live event. For more information or to book an event, contact the Simon & Schuster Speakers Bureau at 1-866-248-3049 or visit our website at www.simonspeakers.com.

Manufactured in China

1   3   5   7   9   10   8   6   4   2

Library of Congress Cataloging-in-Publication Data has been applied for.

ISBN 978-1-6680-2036-4
ISBN 978-1-6680-2037-1 (ebook)

*For my husband, who always encourages
me to dream big and never stops believing in me
even in the moments when I don't believe in myself,
I love you.*

Contents

PART 1
WELCOME (AND GOODBYE) TO THE WEIGHT-LOSS/ HEALTH STALL-OUT STRUGGLE

PART 2

RECIPES FOR DELICIOUS MEALS

CHAPTER 8: Lunch and Dinner

CHAPTER 9: Sauces, Dressings, and Dips

CHAPTER 10: Desserts

ACKNOWLEDGMENTS 246

INDEX 247

Foreword

Dr. Uma Naidoo

We're living in a world where the pursuit of healthy eating feels like a never-ending battlefield of fad diets, quick fixes, and promises of overnight transformations. It's no wonder that many of us have become disillusioned by seemingly unattainable goals set by these diet trends.

And then there's Kiki! In her latest book, *Plantifully Simple: 100 Recipes and Meal Plans for Health and Weight Loss*, she walks us through what she did in her own transformational health journey. Her strategy was not to feel restricted but rather to embrace the many foods she could eat, making her plate *plantiful*, plentiful and delicious while also helping her lose weight.

As we embark on this journey with her, Kiki walks us through part 1 by redefining the numbers game, returning to basic principles, helping us plan a personalized approach, and then providing a 28-day meal plan followed by a maintenance plan. Through the pages of this amazing book, she focuses on the nutritious and delicious elements of embracing more plants. Proven repeatedly in both research and clinical care, more plants in our diet can improve our physical and mental well-being. Her book gives us a glimpse into her world of vibrant health, compassion, and nourishment. Kiki embraces all plant foods and prepares them in a way that enhances their flavor and creates a balance on the plate. Her plan and recipes leave us feeling

there are more food options than less, and there is no restriction—making us feel that this can be sustainable for more people.

The concept of a plant-based diet is not new; in fact, it has been practiced for centuries by various cultures around the world. However, in recent years, as science has caught up with tradition, we have gained a deeper understanding of the profound benefits this way of eating can provide. It's not just about shedding pounds; it's about transforming your relationship with food, optimizing your health, and contributing to a sustainable future for our planet. Embracing plants helps us facilitate weight loss without the feeling of deprivation or endless calorie counting.

Kiki's recipes are bright and delectable—embracing so many plant polyphenols through the colors and textures of the ingredients. Rather than the bland or tasteless meals often assumed to be necessary to support physical health, you'll be introduced to a world of colorful, flavorful, and satisfying dishes. The incredible diversity of plant-based foods ensures that you can enjoy a wide range of flavors and textures while achieving your health and wellness goals. In addition, you are feeding a diversity of nutrients to the extremely key gut microbes that support your overall health. In these pages, you will encounter a wealth of practical advice and strategies to help you on your *plantifully lean* journey.

The type of dietary approach that Kiki writes about is more than a plant-based diet—it is a healthy lifestyle with a deep respect for the environment, and a commitment to personal well-being. When you choose to embrace this way of life, you are not only nourishing your body but also nurturing your soul.

Plants offer a cornucopia of healing properties and a kaleidoscope of colors representing the diverse plant polyphenols and bioactives that can help prevent and manage chronic diseases, boost your immune system, support your mental health, and provide the energy you need to thrive.

As you embark on this book, be prepared for a heartfelt experience of food and recipes that feel like a warm hug from Kiki through her delightful style and presence. She helps us understand that this path is about progress, not perfection. You don't have to make an abrupt transition; you can take gradual steps towards incorporating more plant-based foods into your diet.

As a nutritional psychiatrist focused on the power of food as medicine, I support Kiki's wonderful book as a way to help us on our individual health and wellness journeys.

Dr. Uma Naidoo is a Harvard-trained nutritional psychiatrist, professional chef, nutritional biologist, and author of the bestselling This is Your Brain on Food *and* Calm Your Mind with Food.

PART

1

Welcome (and Goodbye) to the Weight-Loss/Health Stall-Out Struggle

Introduction

Over the past five years, it has been my mission to help as many people as possible connect with their healthiest selves, primarily by shifting how they think about food. Nothing gives me greater joy than seeing them succeed as they learn how to approach their meals as opportunities to change the way they feel.

Several years ago, I embarked on my own weight-loss journey to reclaim my health. Much to my own surprise, I didn't feel trapped by what I *couldn't* eat—rather, I felt liberated by everything I *could* eat. I embraced a diet full of whole, plant-based foods and transformed my health and my body, while also recognizing for the first time the abundance of variety, textures, and flavors, and the straight-up *amount* of food I could eat. My intention has never been to teach people how to "diet," because that implies restriction, frustration, and, ultimately, failure. And I should know: Before discovering this approach to eating, I had been dieting since I was eleven years old.

Like many women, I started becoming aware of my body at a young age. Boys called me chubby. My dieting journey, like that of most people, started with just wanting to lose a little weight because I was teased and I didn't feel happy with the way I looked. But after I gave birth to my daughter, I also needed to address how my body *felt*, because I didn't feel well. I had turned to a low-carbohydrate, high-protein (and therefore high-fat) diet, hoping that it would be a magic path to losing weight quickly. Instead, after several months, I was struggling with hair loss; I was experiencing irregular menstrual cycles and cystic acne as a result of hormonal imbalances that were indicative of polycystic ovarian syndrome; I was prediabetic, with high cholesterol and triglycerides; and I was at increased risk for developing heart disease, the number one cause of death for women.

My doctor's recommendation was to lose quite a bit of weight, and do it *now*. She painted a grim picture of what would happen if I continued to carry this weight: it would put me on a path to chronic disease and a shortened life span.

Attempting to lose five to ten pounds already seemed impossible; how was I supposed to lose more than that?!

Carbs Are Your Friends

Luckily, one of the first distress calls I made was to a friend who told me about Dr. John A. McDougall and his unique approach to nutrition. He was helping people reverse diabetes, heal their bodies, and lose weight by eating…*potatoes*—a food that might as well be the devil to the low-carb community. According to his decades of research and clinical experience, a high-carb, low-fat, plant-based diet was the solution to everything I was struggling with. And more than that, he explained that anyone who was attempting to follow a low-carbohydrate diet over the long term was bound to fail, because the body needs those carbohydrates in order to thrive.

I felt so seen.

I changed my diet immediately. I cut out all animal products (meat, eggs, dairy) and started eating plates full of pasta and potatoes prepared very simply, with just a light spray of oil. It wasn't exactly the most varied diet, but I'm not exaggerating when I say that the weight melted off. In about three months I had lost twenty pounds without even thinking about it. No measuring, no calorie counting, nothing. When I went back to the doctor, she was in disbelief—my cholesterol, triglyceride, and blood sugar levels were all optimal. It was all the proof I needed to continue down this path.

But after months of watching my body and my health transform before my very eyes, I hit the dreaded plateau. Once I lost about twenty-five pounds, I couldn't get another pound to go. And while I had improved my health and my biomarkers were in a much better place, I wanted to continue losing the weight for my health, and would ultimately end up losing seventy pounds. But instead of following the route that so many of us are used to and saying "I'm going to cut out this and that"—which,

after so many years of failed dieting, had become painful and borderline traumatic—I focused on what I could *add* instead. I took a harder look at my pasta- and potato-heavy meals and my cracker and pretzel snacks and thought, *I could probably eat more fruits and vegetables.* I added more of these plants to my plate, and they displaced the processed foods I craved throughout the day. I learned where hidden fats and oils lurked, and I saw the results in how my body looked and felt. I had more energy; I didn't experience the usual afternoon slump; my skin felt hydrated and was less prone to acne; and I was sleeping better and waking up feeling well-rested.

Then, finally, in sight of the goal line, it happened again. My weight loss stalled out. It was tempting to throw in the towel and say that my newfound approach to eating was failing me, but that wouldn't have been entirely true. I felt better, emotionally and physically, than I ever had before, even though I still had a weight-loss goal. I decided to dig even deeper into the question of how food affects the body. My research took me back to the basics: calories in versus calories out. It's the math and the science of health. Did it make me nervous at first, with my years of calorie restriction and driving myself crazy with food logs? You bet.

Liberating Numbers

But I paired this knowledge with something I had never been aware of before, which was the key to my success *and* my peace of mind. It was a concept called "calorie density," or the amount of food in a serving relative to its caloric content.

For example, avocados clock in at 750 calories per pound, whereas a pound of zucchini has 77 calories. That means that, in theory, you could eat almost ten times the amount of zucchini and still have eaten the same number of calories in a pound of avocados. And what's going to satisfy you more—seven pounds of zucchini or one pound of avocados? Not exactly a scenario you'd ever encounter, but you get the idea. Eating more of a food that is less calorie dense will satisfy you.

Instead of seeing these numbers and metrics as oppressive, I learned to see them as the liberating data that they can be—and I learned to make them work for me. Suddenly, I found myself eating *more* food by choosing filling, less calorie-dense options, such as greens and grains, with a sprinkling of more calorie-dense foods, such as sliced avocado, a handful of nuts and seeds, and nondairy dips and dressings. A far cry from the days of Lean Cuisine, when I'd get about half a cup of food per meal and felt hungry for the rest of the day! In addition to a few other simple tweaks that closed the calorie deficit gap—which we'll address in a moment—I was finally able to get that scale to budge. It wasn't that I needed to stop eating a low-fat, plant-based diet; I just needed to put the pieces together in a slightly different way.

Two Paths to Reclaim Your Health

Over the years, I've worked with thousands of people who have come to me and my online wellness programs with the same situation: They want to reclaim their health and lose weight, but feel held back by something they can't figure out. They often had all the information they needed to meet that goal—but they were missing the *tools* for putting it into practice. That's why this book includes tried-and-true strategies that will suit *your* unique objectives, lifestyle, and, most important, relationship with food. These approaches fall into two paths:

Path 1, or Mindfully Plant-Based: Follow a low-fat, plant-based diet using my "balanced plate" method.

Path 2, or Precisely Plant-Based: Follow a low-fat, plant-based diet *and* track your daily calories in order to obtain concrete data for tailoring what you eat to your body's unique needs.

Both paths will deliver results. Both can be a part of your life at one point or another (just as they've both been a part of mine), and both offer freedom and peace of mind when it comes to making food choices.

For many people, simply using my balanced plate method—in which you balance starchy vegetables that satisfy you with fiber-rich, nonstarchy vegetables and don't count macronutrients or calories—is enough to lose weight and maintain results. I rely on this method because I love how effective and liberating this approach to eating is, and I'm happy with where my weight has naturally settled.

For many others, however, reclaiming their health might mean reaching a goal weight that's even more targeted, and being mindful of calories (which we'll talk more about in a bit) can provide the accountability and structure you need for success. That's not because your body works differently from mine or that it's incapable of weight loss—I promise!—it's just that there are many variables when trying to move the scale, and everyone's relationship with food is different.

Those Last Ten Pounds

For example, you may want a more nuanced, detail-oriented approach to weight loss if you're facing what I like to call the Last Ten Pounds. This final bit of weight that you'd like to take off—whether it's actually ten pounds or twelve, seven, or five—can prove to be more stubborn than the weight you lost in the beginning stages of your journey. It was for me! Now, are these pounds the difference between health and chronic disease? For most people, no.

But I get it—you've completely overhauled how you're nourishing yourself, you've most likely transformed your health, and you finally love the way you look and feel, only to hit a wall when it comes to achieving your goals. Frustrating, to say the least! So, while we may call this "vanity weight"—a goal designed more for getting into that swimsuit/dress/pair of skinny jeans than for overall health—I understand that it doesn't make it any less important to you. And because of that, it's important to me.

So long as that goal weight is a healthy one that will support all your body's functions and allow you to live your life to the fullest—something that you need to discuss with your doctor—and so long as you go about losing that weight in a slow, steady way by eating foods that sustain and nourish you, then I'm all in.

The tools you'll find in this book are available for you at any point in your weight-loss journey—from the first ten pounds to the last, and beyond. They're here to offer clarity and reassurance if you've ever felt overwhelmed, anxious, or frustrated by this process. They're here for you whenever you feel like you want to get back to basics and fine-tune your approach to nutrition. Ultimately, this book is your go-to resource for getting the results you deserve after all your hard work, whether it's jump-starting the journey or beating the plateau. I'll give you everything you need to know, in addition to plenty of delicious recipes that will deliver the most food for your calories, with lots of flavor and variety. I'm going to show you how change—and maintenance of that change—is possible with a healthy, plant-based diet and regular low-impact exercise.

No matter how long you've been stuck or yo-yoing, or however many solutions you've tried in the past, I guarantee you that I've got answers. And together, we're finally going to cross that finish line at the end of your weight-loss journey—and keep you on track for a happy, healthy future!

Regardless of whether you're transitioning from a lifetime of eating the Standard American Diet and foods that are high in fat and sugar, or you have a history of struggling with emotional eating, or you've never been able to establish an approach to eating that leads to long-term weight loss, I assure you that you don't have to count a single calorie to be successful.

CHAPTER 1

The Numbers Game

Believe me, I know the frustration—one minute you're cruising along and watching the weight melt off or feeling confident with the new maintenance weight that you and your doctor agree is best for your health, and the next minute you're completely stuck in a rut. That's usually when your mind starts running wild, thinking about all the factors that must be at play—*Is it my age, a medical issue, my exercise, the [fill in the blank] I eat for breakfast every day?* Breaking free from this standstill isn't complicated. It all goes back to Weight Loss 101.

Energy Balance

Let me introduce you to a concept called "energy balance." Energy balance refers to the number of calories your body requires to maintain its current weight. For example, if my body requires 2,000 calories a day to maintain its weight, and I see that my weight hasn't changed, that means that I'm breaking even—I take in and expend those 2,000 calories. This is known as being in energy balance.

Losing weight is a result of eating fewer calories than the daily amount needed to maintain weight. Gaining weight is a result of eating more.

It's simply a numbers game—if you eat fewer calories than your body needs to maintain its weight, you lose weight. Now, I know what you're thinking right now:

There's no way I'm eating too much.

I eat perfectly and never have any treats.

I work out like crazy.

It must be my thyroid/age/menopause.

I've heard it all, and I've helped thousands of people with each of these circumstances reach their goals. All these individuals have been different ages, weights, nationalities, and ethnicities, and they've all had different medical issues. I was a hypothyroid patient at the beginning of my weight-loss journey. And while there are definitely some physiological factors that can play a role in not being able to lose weight easily, **I'm here to encourage you to embrace the idea that, most likely, there is nothing sneaky going on here. It's simply the numbers.**

Plant-Based Diets Create a Calorie Deficit

When you're just beginning your weight-loss journey or have a lot of weight to lose, creating a calorie deficit can be pretty straightforward—meaning it's easier to consume fewer calories than your body needs, especially if you switch to eating wholesome, plant-based foods that are full of water, fiber, bulk, and nutrients that keep you feeling satisfied all day long: foods such as broccoli, zucchini, melons, apples, berries, potatoes, and whole grains such as oats, rice, and quinoa. These foods also happen to be dramatically lower in calories than animal-based foods, which is why you're able to eat more food than ever before yet still lose weight.

But when you get closer to your body's ideal weight—meaning a weight that's within the ideal range your doctor determines based on your age, sex, height, and ethnicity—it can be trickier to consistently create a calorie deficit. That's because by losing weight, you've narrowed the gap between the calories you're taking in and the calorie deficit needed to support weight loss. So even if you're doing everything "right"—you're eating a low-fat diet full of a variety of fruits and vegetables and getting plenty of regular exercise—your body has settled into a new energy balance with the number of calories you're currently eating. And when that happens, the window for creating a calorie deficit without inducing drastic hunger becomes smaller.

But here's the good news: When you're consistently eating foods that contain 650 calories per pound or fewer (i.e., most plant-based foods and no animal products; see page 12 for a list), as well as following my plate-building method (page 15), **you will naturally create a deficit that puts your body in a healthy energy balance.** (And without requiring intense physical activity, too—but more on that in a bit.) Regardless of whether you're transitioning from a lifetime of eating the Standard American Diet and foods that are high in fat and sugar, or you have a history of struggling with emotional eating, or

you've never been able to establish an approach to eating that leads to long-term weight loss, I assure you that if you eat the foods on page 12 without counting a single calorie, you will be successful.

When you're eating a low-fat, whole-food, plant-based diet, your appetite will naturally help you consume the number of calories you need to reach and sustain a healthy weight. That's because the amount of low-fat, plant-based foods you need to eat in order to feel full and satisfied is always going to be lower in calories than processed or animal foods. And when at last you can trust your body's cues about fullness and not have to worry about trying to outsmart your biofeedback signals in the name of not gaining weight, then you can finally step off the dangerous binge-and-restrict cycle and embrace the peace of mind that comes with knowing you can eat without restriction and still lose weight. You don't have to look any further than nature to see this in action.

Wild animals maintain optimal weights because they're eating only the food nature designed for them, and their appetites make sure they get just enough and not too much. The only animals you see with weight problems are humans and animals who live with humans, especially cats and dogs. That's because we've stepped away from nature's optimal food sources and are instead eating animal foods and processed foods that are high in fat and sugar. But when we return to the whole, low-fat, plant-based foods we were meant to thrive on, our bodies automatically know how to calibrate, ensuring our best chance of health and survival.

But nature can sometimes also complicate

this process. Another reason that losing weight is difficult is because your body is trying to protect you. Your body is designed to weather the lean seasons people endured thousands of years ago when food was hard to come by; it retains fat to protect your organs, keep you warm, and fuel your brain—in other words, to survive!

Women's bodies evolved to store fat in order to ensure that we can maintain the energy stores we need to support pregnancies, especially during times when food is scarce. In fact, researchers have found that not only are women predisposed to carry more body fat but our bodies are also specifically programmed to *not* lose weight, even with calorie-burning efforts such as exercise and dietary calorie deficits.[1]

What does all this add up to? It explains why losing weight isn't easy, even if you're carrying more weight than is advisable. Our bodies evolved to store fat—so if you've struggled with weight loss in the past, know that it doesn't mean there's something wrong with you or that you're a failure. It's nature. Thankfully, there are ways to healthfully encourage your body to let go of the reins just enough to get the results you're looking for.

---

1   John A. McDougall, MD, *The McDougall Program for Maximum Weight Loss* (New York: Penguin, 1995), 81–84.

CHAPTER 2

Getting Back to Basics

I f you're going to be successful in reaching your goal weight—and I know you will be!—then you're going to have to take things back to the basics of calories. I know that this can be unnerving to those of you who've had a complicated relationship with the C word, but understanding how calories work in the body—even if you choose not to actively track how many you eat in a day—is crucial. And I promise that we're going after this in a new way that's about liberation, not restriction—meaning you'll be able to eat more to weigh less. That all begins with understanding calorie density.

Calorie Density

Calorie density is a simple measure of energy (calories) in any given weight of food—which, for our purposes, will be in calories per pound. So, to use the example I cited earlier, there are 750 calories in one pound of avocados and 77 calories in one pound of zucchini. You want the bulk of your meals to be made up of foods that are *lowest* in calorie density, because that means you get more food on your plate for fewer calories.

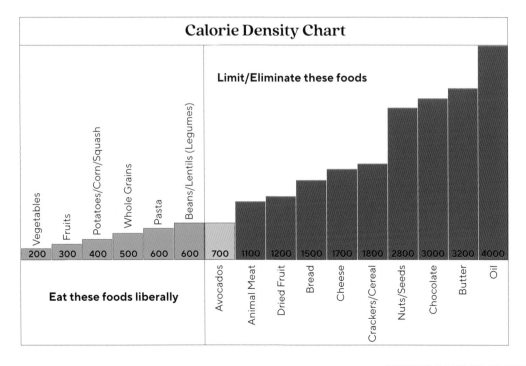

What Keeps You Satisfied?

It also happens that the foods that are lowest in calorie density are also the foods that are highest in nutrition, water, fiber, and bulk, because they haven't been dehydrated, combined with preservatives, or processed. When foods are processed, the water, fiber, and bulk are removed, usually so they can survive longer in a package. Then, in order to make these foods irresistible to consumers, food manufacturers add salt, sugar, and/or fat. Processed foods are almost always less filling than their unprocessed versions, and they are certainly higher in calorie density. Here's an example:

If you eat two large apples, you will have consumed around two hundred calories. You will reap the benefits of the apple's natural water, fiber, and nutrition, and you'll feel pretty full. By contrast, if you eat two hundred calories' worth of dried apples, you'll get the same vitamins and minerals, but because the apples have been stripped of their natural water content—which is part of what helps signal to the brain that the body has had enough to eat—it won't satisfy you. What often happens is that we just reach for more dried apples until our stomach signals to our brain that it's had enough—after having consumed significantly more food (and, therefore, calories) to reach the same level of satiety. I'm not saying that dried apples aren't healthy—they're just a more calorically dense option than a whole apple.

You need to eat many more dried apples than fresh apples to feel full.

Whether you want to lose weight or maintain the weight you've lost, you want to build your meals using foods that have 650 calories per pound or fewer. All other plant-based foods should be eaten in moderation, especially when it comes to losing the last few pounds.

How Foods Fill the Belly (or Don't)

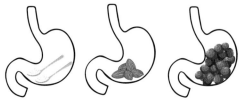

2 Tbsp Vegetable Oil
240 calories

1/4 Cup Almonds
240 calories

5 Cups Strawberries
240 calories

FOODS LOWEST IN CALORIE DENSITY

Greens (lettuce, kale, spinach, arugula):
100 calories per pound

Nonstarchy vegetables (cucumbers, mushrooms, celery, zucchini, onions, broccoli, cauliflower, tomatoes, asparagus, Brussels sprouts, cabbage, bok choy):
200 calories per pound

Fresh fruit (apples, oranges, berries, melons, peaches, pears, grapes, pineapples):
300 calories per pound

Starchy vegetables (white potatoes, sweet potatoes, corn, butternut squash, acorn squash, carrots, pumpkin):
400 to 500 calories per pound

Whole grains (oats, rice, millet, barley, quinoa):
550 calories per pound

Beans and lentils:
600 calories per pound

FOODS HIGHEST IN CALORIE DENSITY

Avocados:
750 calories per pound

Breads, bagels, wraps:
1,400 calories per pound

Dry cereal and cheese:
1,500 calories per pound

Crackers and processed sugar:
1,800 calories per pound

Chocolate and potato chips:
2,500 calories per pound

Nuts, seeds, and butters:
2,800 calories per pound

Oils:
4,000 calories per pound

Also consider that pork, beef, chicken, fish, eggs, and ice cream are all around 1,200 calories per pound—yet another reason to follow a plant-based diet!

Eating Plants Activates Weight Loss

In addition to naturally *aiding* weight loss because of their low calorie density, plants also actively *interact* with our body's composition to *encourage* weight loss.

The research of Dr. William Li, the *New York Times* bestselling author of *Eat to Beat Disease* and *Eat to Beat Your Diet*, shows that certain plant-derived compounds affect how fat is stored in the body. For example, lycopene, which is found in foods such as tomatoes, car-

Free Calories

Because nonstarchy vegetables are so low in calories, whenever you add **1 cup or less** to your meals or to one of my recipes, I consider them "free" calories. Meaning that regardless of whether you fill a chickpea omelet with onions, spinach, and mushrooms or bell peppers and tomatoes, you won't need to worry about calculating every last calorie because the difference is negligible. That's also why these vegetables make such great snacks along with more calorie-dense dips and dressings; you're taking in fewer calories but more food volume, which we'll talk about in more detail on pages 15–16.

rots, watermelon, and grapefruit, breaks down fat cells, and ingredients such as turmeric, ginseng, and broccoli can suppress the growth of fat cells (as well as deprive cancer cells of nourishment). Similarly, there are plants that have the power to fire up brown fat, the paper-thin sheath of fat that encloses your muscles, organs, and bones and whose purpose is to regulate your body temperature. When activated, brown fat can burn calories, control blood sugar, and dissolve white fat molecules (otherwise known as the "squishy" fat that we're often trying to get rid of).

In people who have more body fat overall, brown fat is often not activated. But, according to Dr. Li, certain foods trigger the release of norepinephrine, a neurotransmitter that helps regulate your mood and your sleep-wake cycle, and that "switches on" your brown fat cells (via what's called beta-3 adrenergic receptors).[1]

Eating Plants Boosts Your Mood

Yet another benefit of eating a diet rich in plants is that they can improve how you feel not just physically but also mentally. Dr. Uma Naidoo, author of *This Is Your Brain on Food*, has dedicated her research to the mood-food connection. After years of treating patients and investigating how to better help them cope with depression, anxiety, and even PTSD and ADHD through a combination of diet and medication, she observed that the food we eat has a direct effect on our mood and mindset.

Unsurprisingly, the food we eat changes the types of bacteria present in our gut microbiome. What Dr. Naidoo has shown, however, is that when our gut is well nourished with beneficial bacteria, we are more likely to feel content and uplifted. That's because the gut and brain are directly connected by the vagus nerve, which carries signals between the two parts of the body. When our gut is out of balance and there's an overgrowth of bad bacteria (often as a result of eating processed foods), our brain signals are also off-kilter, and we can feel depressed and strained.

This gut-brain connection is just one of many reasons why eating for optimal gut health is so important. But what's the number one driver of gut health? You guessed it: plants. Specifically, plants with **probiotic** and **prebiotic** qualities. Probiotic foods contribute beneficial bacteria to the gut, and prebiotic foods contain certain types of fiber that the beneficial bacteria in our gut digest, keeping them fed and happy. Below is a list of probiotic and prebiotic foods, many of which you will find in my recipes.

FOODS THAT HELP BURN CALORIES	GREAT SOURCES OF PROBIOTICS	GREAT SOURCES OF PREBIOTICS
Apples	Kimchi	Apples
Berries	Kombucha	Bananas
Coffee	Miso	Barley
Cranberries	Sauerkraut	Cocoa
Grapefruit	Tempeh	Flaxseeds
Grapes	Yogurt (I like coconut yogurt)	Garlic
Green Tea		Jerusalem artichokes
Hot peppers		Leeks
Leafy Greens		Legumes
Lentils		Oats
Oats		Onions
Whole Grains		Seaweed

---

1   William W. Li, MD, *Eat to Beat Your Diet: Burn Fat, Heal Your Metabolism, and Live Longer* (New York: Balance, 2023), 81–87

Diluting Calories, Satiety, and Preloading Your Meals

In addition to taking in fewer calories by reaching for less calorie-dense foods, other strategies for reducing your caloric intake are diluting your calories and "preloading" your meals. These strategies are applicable to both of the paths I'll describe later in this book.

Preloading simply means eating foods in a sequence that puts the most filling foods first.

Diluting is a way to visualize how much of your plate you'll fill with different types of foods in order to ensure that what you're eating will meet your nutrient and calorie goals. The 50/50 plate is a great example.

My various plate-building methods make use of these strategies to help you lose weight without counting calories, no matter where you are in your weight-loss journey.

Starting with the 50/50 Plate

This is the best place to begin when you're first wrapping your head around getting the most mileage out of your calories, regardless of whether you're counting them.

Visualize a dinner plate filled with something delicious and plant-based; let's say steamed potatoes with 1 cup of Pimento Cheese Sauce (page 225). Yum! That's a total of six hundred calories. Then imagine a line going down the middle of your plate; on one half you still have your cheesy potatoes, but on the other, replace the potatoes that were there with a nonstarchy vegetable—let's say steamed broccoli. That broccoli is only one hundred calories, which

means you've just shaved two hundred calories off your plate but none of the volume.

> ### If You Just Do One Thing, Cut Back on Oil
>
> The foundation of my approach to living a happy, healthy, satisfied life in a body that reflects your true beauty inside and out is eating a diet composed of foods that contain 650 calories per pound or fewer. If I could choose just one change for you to make in order to see results, it would be to cut back on how much oil you're using in your meals, if not cut it out entirely.
>
> Oil is *the* most calorie-dense food on the planet, and it adds unnecessary amounts of fat and calories to your meals, whether you're cooking with it, drizzling it on finished dishes, or buying products that contain it. Think of it this way: You can keep the oil, but you're going to have to limit a ton of other foods to compensate for all the tasteless calories you're taking in. And that oil is not filling your belly. To me, it's just not worth it—especially when you see how easy it is to prepare delicious, creamy sauces and dressings without a drop of oil. But if you're still not convinced or want to ease yourself into this transition, you can add a light coating of avocado oil cooking spray to your pan when sautéing.

It's something I like to call **diluting your calories**, and it's a clear way to see how you can eat lots of food and still lose weight.

The broccoli, or any nonstarchy veggie you love, not only helps bring the calorie count down but also adds more bulk and weight to help trigger a feeling of *satiety*, or feeling full.

While popular diet culture tells us that protein and fat trigger satiety, research proves that's not the case. In one study, researchers asked participants to eat plates full of oil-free pasta with fat-free marinara. They then had people report how full they felt and how long it was until they felt hungry again. For their next meal, participants were given the same plates of pasta, but this time drizzled with oil instead of the marinara. What they found was that the oil had no effect on participants' feelings of satiety or how long those feelings lasted. It also didn't help them eat less. The researchers were therefore able to conclude that it was the weight of the food consumed and the volume it took up in the stomach that had the biggest effect on satiety. And whole, plant-based foods below the six-hundred-calorie-per-pound mark just happen to have the most volume and fiber, and are also the heaviest, owing to their water content.

The Benefit of Starchy Foods

Now, don't go thinking that you can outsmart your body and live on lettuce and cucumbers alone. You would be hungry—and that might make you grouchy and irritable and leave you wanting to throw in the towel. That's where those starchy foods come in. The calories from things like whole grains, starchy vegetables,

and legumes also have the fiber to fill you up and keep you feeling sated for a while. So, when you pair wholesome starches with nonstarchy vegetables, you have the perfect weight-loss combination . . . which brings me back to that 50/50 equation you can use as a starting point for building all your meals (and that's echoed in most of the recipes in this book): a plate **half filled with nonstarchy vegetables and half filled with starches of your choice that have been prepared without oil or with just a light spray.**

Eat Your Vegetables First

Preloading your meal means first eating the foods that are high in fiber and bulk but low in calorie density so that you will start to feel full earlier in the meal. It's really just a fancy way of saying you should start your meal with vegetables—such as in a soup or a salad—before moving on to your main course. I've given you a basic recipe for how to build a preloading salad or soup on page 190. This will help you fill up on less calorie-dense foods before eating the more calorie-dense part of your meal.

Graduating from the 50/50 Plate to the Lean Plate

Even if you choose the weight-loss path that includes tracking calories, I still want you to learn elements of the plate-building method, because it can be a powerful guide for building meals and never having to guess at what to eat.

It's also helpful if you're eating in a restaurant or at someone else's home.

If you've been using the 50/50 plate and are feeling good but your weight loss is stalling out or getting more difficult because you're closing in on your weight-loss goal, that's where the **Lean Plate** comes in. This plate is half filled with nonstarchy vegetables, one-quarter filled with a starch, and the remaining quarter filled with fruit. You're reducing the number of higher-calorie foods on your plate but replacing them with high-volume, high-fiber foods that will hit the satiety mark. When sitting down to eat, I recommend starting with your nonstarchy vegetables so that you fill up on the

The Lean Plate

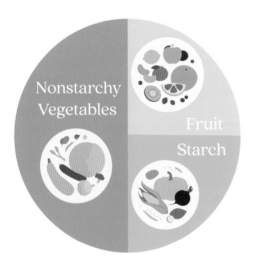

least calorie-dense foods with the highest nutrition. And if you're still hungry after eating everything on your plate, fill a second plate the exact same way and start with your nonstarchy vegetables once again! Be consistent at every meal and you'll be well on your way to meeting your goals.

Will I Feel Deprived?

The most surprising truth I discovered on my own weight-loss journey was this: You can enjoy delicious meals and desserts that feel decadent and satisfying *and* lose weight! It's all about learning to make over your favorite foods in ways that leave behind the weight-gain-promoting fats and oils and unhealthy processed ingredients in favor of whole, plant-based foods. When I was losing weight, I knew that if I couldn't enjoy the pancakes, waffles, pizza, and egg rolls that made me happy, then this lifestyle wasn't going to be sustainable for me. That's when I started experimenting with recipes that delivered the same flavors and textures as the foods I loved. If your meals don't satisfy you—physically or emotionally—then it's just another diet. And all diets fail.

I created the recipes in this book so that you can not only achieve your health and weight-loss goals but also do it in a way that's enjoyable. What's more, when you enjoy eating these foods and genuinely look forward to your meals, then these changes become habits. And those habits add up to a sustainable, pleasurable, happy-making lifestyle.

Will Eating Fewer Calories Ruin or Slow Down My Metabolism?

One of the and most enduring falsehoods about weight loss is that if you diet or restrict your calories, then your metabolism is going to slow down.

Think of it this way: Suppose that, in order to maintain your original weight, you were eating 2,000 calories a day. You then reduced your calories to 1,800 a day, and your weight went down. So now, eating 1,800 calories a day is going to maintain that new weight. Nothing has changed in your metabolism; your body has just adjusted to a new energy balance. If, however, you start eating more than 1,800 calories a day, your weight will go up. So, when anyone comes to me saying they believe their metabolism isn't kicking in the way it's supposed to or they're having a difficult time losing weight—or they're constantly gaining weight—especially toward the end of their weight-loss journey, I say the same thing: Have you tried a consistent caloric deficit? That's right—the very program I'm recommending here is what will help your body nudge its way past that plateau, metabolism and all.

Why Am I Not Tracking Macros?

Macronutrients—fats, carbohydrates, and proteins—are the building blocks of everything you eat, and tracking macronutrients is simply the process of adding up the grams of fat, carbohydrates, and protein in your meals throughout the day to make sure you're hitting the optimal ratio for the purposes of weight loss or muscle gain. I believe tracking macros is cumbersome and makes people worry about how much protein, fat, and carbohydrates they're consuming.

You absolutely do not have to track macros to lose weight. In fact, many of the recommendations for "ideal" macro ratios are protein-heavy and full of fat. Instead, by following a low-fat, high-carbohydrate, plant-based diet, your body will naturally get the calories and the nutrition it needs, and in the right ratios. However, I understand that this idea is new to a lot of people, so I've included this section to explain why I'm not so concerned about monitoring every last gram of protein, fat, and carbohydrates.

Protein

The diet industry markets the idea that you need an abundance of protein to lose weight and gain muscle. This helps them create demand for expensive protein bars, drinks, and powders. Case in point: What's the first question you get when you tell people that you eat a plant-based diet? *Where do you get your protein?* This is the number one question I'm asked when people are considering switching to a plant-based lifestyle. It was also one of my main concerns until I started reading books and attending lectures given by prominent physicians such as Dr. Neal Barnard, Dr. John McDougall, and Dr. Michael Klaper. The idea that we could be protein deficient is just a fallacy. When was the last time you heard of someone being diagnosed with a "protein deficiency"? I never have, and that's because true protein deficiencies only occur where famine and starvation are present, causing severe malnutrition.

We can find all the protein we need in whole plants. Plants are a rich source of complete proteins and amino acids (the building blocks of complete proteins) and meet all the protein requirements of some of the world's largest animals, such as elephants, gorillas, cows, and hippopotamuses. Forty to sixty grams of protein a day is more than anybody needs, and that's drastically lower than the one hundred grams or more a day that we're told we need by so-called health companies that want to sell us products with additional sources of protein.

Fat

Fat is another heavily marketed nutrient that, like protein, we need less of than big food companies tell us in their marketing. Companies that produce cheese, nut butters, and cooking oils want you to believe that you require their products for your health.

Our bodies don't require any additional fat. Not only is your body *very* efficient at storing it (see page 9 for a refresher on why) but fat is also not your body's preferred fuel source—carbohydrates are. Only 7 percent of the fat you ingest goes toward vital functions, such as making new cells and manufacturing hormones. But that leaves 93 percent that isn't required for anything. Any guesses as to where it goes? Yep—your tissues. It gets stored there in case your energy needs aren't being met by carbohydrates, and as I said before, your body is very good at planning for emergencies. What's also worth thinking about is that the fat itself doesn't have to be converted to another form before it's stored. In other words, when you eat fat, that fat is stored as-is in your body.

Plant foods—even lettuce!—contain trace amounts of fat, but nature perfectly combines that fat with fiber, water, and micronutrients so our bodies can use it. When just the oil is extracted from plants, you're left with a highly processed, highly fattening and calorically dense product (this is true even of olive and avocado oils), so it's best to use these sources of fat sparingly. Rest easy knowing that you're getting enough fat from all the plants you eat. Avocados, nuts, and seeds contain wonderful nutrients and make tasty additions to your meals, in moderation.

Carbohydrates

Unprocessed carbohydrates from foods like potatoes, rice, beans, and oats will not make you fat. Those foods are low in fat and calories and are extremely filling, making them perfect weight-loss foods. I lost seventy pounds eating carbs, after years of unsuccessfully following low-carb diets. The carbs that *are* fattening are the ones processed with fat and sugar—foods such as potato chips, crackers, cereal, and, of course, classic junk food like doughnuts and cookies. Carbohydrates are satisfying, and you can find that bliss in foods like potatoes (my favorite), rice, farro, beans and other legumes, oats, and corn. While the bulk of your calories should come from unprocessed sources, because that's the best way to eat more and weigh less, it's appropriate to make room for some processed foods, such as low-calorie, whole-grain products like wraps and breads. It's another great way to enjoy eating carbs while still being able to reach your goals.

CHAPTER 3

Tailoring
It to You

The weight-loss journey is far from a one-size-fits-all experience. Everything from your genetic constitution to your relationship with food to your preference for structure versus something a little more go-with-the-flow informs what kind of approach will be most effective for forming healthy new habits. Both approaches to losing weight are highly effective and appropriate for all individuals. But the one you pick needs to work for *you*. It needs to feel right. And, most important, it needs to feel enjoyable and satisfying.

Choosing Your Path

What I love most about having two paths to weight loss is that it can change as your needs change. If you're just starting out and have been enjoying being Mindfully Plant-Based but are curious about being Precisely Plant-Based, try it out for a week! Or maybe you've noticed that your weight has been creeping up during your maintenance phase (which we'll talk more about in Chapter 6) and you want to go back to a solid baseline. Maybe you've gotten great results with a more targeted approach and want a little less structure for a period of time. Whatever your reasoning, these paths and their tools are here for you.

Path 1: Mindfully Plant-Based

This is the most basic model, or what I like to call "simply eating plants." There isn't much more to do here than reach for low-fat, plant-based foods as you use the plate-building method from page 15. If it sounds too good to be true, I assure you that it most certainly is not! This path is perfect for individuals who are just starting out on their journey back to health or are new to plant-based eating; anyone who prefers not to track calories; and those who have reached their weight-loss goal using Path 2 and want to maintain their success without tracking calories.

To start on this path, skip ahead to page 27 for tools that will help you build strong new habits. Or take a peek at the recipes on page 47 to start getting excited about all the options for this week's meals.

Path 2:
Precisely Plant-Based

This is what I think of as a more targeted approach to weight loss. You'll still be following a low-fat, plant-based diet, but with the addition of tracking calories. The goal is still to feel satisfied and full after every meal and between meals, but the biggest difference between this and the Mindfully Plant-Based path is that you'll see exactly how many calories you're taking in each day. This approach is ideal for people who aren't seeing the results they want using the more open-ended path and need to make sure they're staying within a deficit range, those who want a more structured approach to their meals, and people who are motivated by hard data. There's a little more setup than with Path 1, but once you've completed the following steps, you won't have to expend much more effort.

Step 1: Find your energy balance, or the number of calories your body needs to sustain its current weight. To do this, I recommend an online total daily energy expenditure (TDEE) calculator. This calculator helps you assess your caloric needs by taking into account your gender, age, height, weight, body fat percentage, and current activity level. It will show you the number of calories you need to maintain your current weight, as well as to lose weight. For example, you can use the calculator to generate the optimal number of calories to eat if you want to lose one pound a week.

My favorite version of this calculator can be found at tdeecalculator.net.

Step 2: Choose the correct activity multi-plier. I don't know how many times I've heard from frustrated and defeated individuals who tell me they do everything right—eat right, track every single thing they eat, exercise regularly, get plenty of sleep—only to see that they've made a simple mistake: They pick an activity level that's too high for them. (Most people *underestimate* the number of calories they're taking in and *overestimate* the amount of daily activity they get.) As a result, many people adjust their calorie needs to a higher activity level, which often results in a plateau or, in some cases, weight gain. This happens because we often think we're more active than we actually are. Whether you're troubleshooting or checking that you're doing everything right, it's essential that you choose the correct activity multiplier, because doing so will ensure that you're taking in the appropriate number of calories for your activity level, and also not deducting too many calories for exercise you aren't getting.

The calculators themselves can be misleading, so here's what to consider when choosing an activity setting using a TDEE calculator:

To help you answer the activity-level question on a TDEE calculator, consider the following:

1. Sedentary: Fewer than three thousand steps a day, spending most of your day sitting. Daily activities include shopping, cleaning, walking the dog, and mowing the lawn.
2. Lightly Active: Three thousand to ten thousand steps a day (four miles); spending twenty to thirty minutes a day doing vigorous activity such as aerobics, running, or biking; or spending a good portion of your day on your feet (salesperson, teacher).

3. Active: Ten thousand to twenty-three thousand steps a day (four to ten miles); getting one hour of intense exercise every day; or spending a good part of the day doing some physical activity (restaurant server, hospital nurse, mail carrier).
4. Athlete: More than twenty-three thousand steps a day; two hours of intense exercise every day, such as running; or spending most of the day doing heavy physical activity (carpenter, furniture mover, bike messenger).

When to Adjust Your Daily Caloric Limit

I caution people to not cut more than five hundred calories a day. Creating a larger deficit than that will likely leave you feeling dissatisfied, cranky, and hungry, and that often leads to binging.

A two hundred to five hundred calorie deficit is not so drastic that it's unsustainable or unhealthy. A 250-calorie-a-day deficit will prompt a weekly loss of half a pound, and a 500-calorie-a-day deficit will prompt a weekly loss of one pound, provided that you're maintaining a consistent deficit in these amounts. You may need to play with this number until you find the right one for you.

While you may initially experience some hunger when adjusting to a plant-based diet and consuming fewer calories—especially if you're used to eating a lot of animal foods—I don't want you to feel dissatisfied all the time. If that's the case, consider increasing your daily calorie allotment. The other reason to readust

your daily caloric limit is if you've lost five to ten pounds. At this point it's a good idea to recalibrate, because your body has most likely adjusted to your deficit. Running the numbers again using your updated weight will give you a more accurate caloric limit.

Tracking Calories

Tracking calories is merely a tool. It does *not* need to be done forever. (Do you keep hammer-

The Third Path

As you'll read more about in Chapter 6, there is actually a third path, what I call the **Maintenance Path**. I designed this path for individuals who have reached their goal weight and no longer need to sustain a calorie deficit, but it can also be a great option *before* you've gotten to that point. On the Maintenance Path, you have more flexibility regarding the amount and types of food you eat, because you're merely maintaining your weight instead of actively trying to lose weight. As a result, it can be a nice reprieve if you find yourself wanting to take a step away from your current weight-loss path without derailing your progress. It's also a great tool for navigating occasions when it's more difficult to plan or prepare your meals, such as vacations and holidays.

ing a nail once it's lodged in the wall? No. You put the hammer away.)

Calorie counting will help you internalize the amount of food you need to lose or maintain weight. If tracking calories helps you feel comfortable with your food choices, then do it for as long as you want. I've found that most people like to track calories, and those who do track them—even loosely—are the most successful at reaching their weight-loss goals. As the old saying goes, "What you don't measure, you can't control."

Also, for many people, counting calories can give them a feeling of food freedom. They're able to see how much food they can actually eat and still lose weight. That's a pleasant surprise; they feel hope and don't feel restricted.

Some people find it comforting to know exactly how much fuel they're putting in compared to how much they're burning. If you look at calorie counting as just a way to collect data and not as a way to restrict yourself, then it can be an extremely useful tool that will work well for you.

Choosing a Calorie Tracker

There are many free online calorie trackers with additional upgrades available for purchase. Of these, I like Cronometer, which has a huge database of foods and their calorie information. You can also enter your own custom recipes and save your favorite items so that your daily entries are quick and easy. Similarly, you can download MyFitnessPal and use it in essentially the same way.

Weighing Your Food

It's one thing to tally the calories you eat; it's another to make sure you're getting an *accurate* tally. A pitfall I frequently see is when people measure their food in cups or tablespoons rather than by weight. A medium potato might look different to you than it does to the next person, but there can be a 150- to 200-calorie difference between them. That can account for 10 percent of your calories. Weighing your food eliminates uncertainty and makes for much more accurate accounting of your caloric intake.

I've included weight measures in my recipes for the ingredients where it makes the biggest difference—mainly potatoes, rice, beans, corn, oats, peanut butter, nuts, avocados, and bananas. However, there are some ingredients for which you won't see weights—such as fruits, vegetables, greens, dressings, and liquids—since the caloric difference would be negligible.

If weighing your food becomes an obstacle or a deterrent, you can skip this step. Eat with enjoyment and faith that my recipes are designed to help you meet your weight-loss goals.

Keeping a Food Journal

Keeping a food journal will help you create new and sustainable habits. First, it will give you an extreme sense of satisfaction as you fill out the last entry for the day, even if your meals weren't your best choices. Why? Because you're connecting with yourself and the things you're doing to bring yourself better health or joy or pride. The individuals I've worked with who keep food journals are, hands down, more successful not only in getting the weight off but in keeping it off as well. Here is an example of what I eat in a day and how I record my entries:

$\mathcal{Day}$ 0

DATE: 01/01/2021 BED TIME: 9:30 WAKE TIME: 5:30 HOURS SLEPT: 8 hrs

BREAKFAST	LUNCH	DINNER	WATER
Blueberry Pancakes w/	Baked Fries/Ketchup	Burrito Bowl w/ Avocado	◇ ◇
1 Tbsp maple syrup	Roasted Brussel Sprouts	Salad w/ Vegan Ranch	◇ ◇
Steamed Asparagus	Bowl of Berries		◇ ◇
			◇ ◇

OUNCES
64 oz

SNACKS
Orange slices, frozen cherries

Did I enjoy my daily movement?

☒ yes - loved it
☐ eh - not so much

How do I feel about it?

① ② ③ ④ ⑤ ⑥ ⑦ ⑧ ⑨ ⊗

Write something I appreciate about my body/self.
I appreciate my body's ability to adapt and change

Did I love myself today with my food and movement choices?

① ② ③ ④ ⑤ ⑥ ⑦ ⑧ ⑨ ⊗

How can I love myself more tomorrow?
I will compliment myself more tomorrow.

Dos and Don'ts of Creating a Calorie Deficit

Don't reduce your caloric intake so much that you set yourself up to fail.

Reduce your calories by two hundred to five hundred a day; a greater cut may cause you to feel so ravenously hungry that you end up eating far more food than you need. (Which is why I suggest you use the simple method developed by researchers at Harvard that's laid out to the right if you're within five to ten pounds of your goal weight.)

Your hunger drive is completely normal and healthy—nature made it that way to make sure you provide your body with the fuel it needs. So being hungry is nothing to be ashamed of or ignored. The key is to create a relationship with your hunger so you can hear what it really needs, and then satisfy that hunger with the best food choices possible (ideally foods that are low in fat and calorie density).

If you're restricting your calories too extremely because you believe that if a little is good, then more is better, you're going to risk kicking your hunger drive into high gear. When that happens, your body hits the panic button, which in turn sends your brain signals that you need to eat anything that isn't nailed down. A moderate deficit (of two hundred to five hundred calories a day), however, will help you lose weight while also keeping your hunger cues calibrated.

Another Simple Way to Determine Your Caloric Needs

If you're within fifteen pounds of your goal weight and want an even easier way to calculate your caloric needs, regardless of your activity level, try the method below, which was developed by researchers at Harvard.

For Weight Loss

Multiply your goal weight by twelve to establish your daily caloric limit.

For example: If your goal weight is 140 pounds, multiply 140 by twelve, which equals 1,680. That's going to be your daily caloric limit to reach your goal weight of 140 pounds.

For Weight Maintenance

Multiply your weight by fifteen.

So, if you reach your goal weight of 140 pounds, multiply that by fifteen, which equals 2,100. This will be your daily caloric limit to maintain your weight.

Don't try to eat too perfectly.

Eating a "perfect" diet is straight-up impossible. At some point, you will give in and have a little (or a lot) of whatever food it is you're trying to avoid. Then comes the guilt and shame cycle. First, I want you to promise yourself to never feel guilty or ashamed about food again. These are damaging and counterproductive feelings, and no food should make you feel emotionally bad. Second, I want you to realize that you can

Be Honest with Yourself

Just as many people have a difficult time accurately assessing how active they are during the day, the same thing happens when it comes to how much they're eating. Some people think they're eating less than they actually are, even when they're tracking calories. They may not count the little handful of nuts here or the three crackers there—but these small, untracked grabs can add up to an *additional* two hundred to four hundred calories a day, which makes weight loss impossible—especially when they're trying to create a two-hundred- to five-hundred-calorie daily deficit.

The weekend is also a common blind spot. I see it all the time—someone feels like they're being good all week, so they sneak in some extra indulgences over the weekend. But the key to breaking through a weight-loss plateau is maintaining a *consistent* calorie deficit. So, if you're watching every calorie during the week only to exceed your deficit during the weekend, you're not going to get the desired results. In fact, many people end up gaining weight and undoing all the hard work they're putting in Monday through Friday! This is why it's important to plan for your weekend meals as well as your weekday meals, in addition to finding foods that you enjoy so much that it doesn't feel like you're missing out on your favorite treats.

make room for the foods you love, especially if you work on finding lower-calorie versions of them. It's essential that you make this journey an enjoyable one so that it can also be a sustainable one. The people I work with who try to be the most perfect are always the first ones to burn out or feel out of control when confronted by the foods they love most.

Remember: balance is key, and it will look different for each of us.

Do eat the foods you enjoy.

Just because you're placing some parameters on what you eat (e.g., sticking with foods with low calorie density) doesn't mean that you need to force yourself to eat things you don't like. Hate kale? Don't eat it! Can't stand oats? Leave 'em alone! There are *plenty* of other plants out there to choose from. A big part of my success was finding ways to be able to enjoy pizza, waffles, and chocolate without undermining my progress. Find the veggies and meals you enjoy and eat them on repeat. You're already challenging yourself; you might as well make it easier!

Tips for Making a Calorie Deficit Not Feel Like a Deficit

One of the best ways to be successful on your weight-loss journey is to keep your calorie deficit from feeling like a deficit at all. You can do this in several ways:

1. **Eat high-volume foods.** Choose whole, plant-based foods—as in, foods that look as close as possible to how they grow in nature. These foods are full of water, bulk, fiber, and nutrients that help you fill up and keep you feeling satisfied. Instead of snacking on one cup of potato chips for two hundred calories, eat two medium potatoes for two hundred calories. It will be much more filling than the chips. Here are more examples of easy tips:

2. **Eat dinner (or a snack) later so that you avoid pre-bedtime binging.** There's this idea out there that "if you eat after eight, you will gain weight," but that's not true. Many nutritionists have, in fact, confirmed that eating later in the day—regardless of what kind of diet you're following—does not lead to weight gain. Eating too many calories, however, does—as does eating too much fat and salt, which will lead to water retention. But could you eat only doughnuts before bed if you were in a calorie deficit and still lose weight? Technically, yes. (Although I don't recommend it!) So that's why eating your last meal later can be a great secret weapon for feeling satiated all day.

   I like to eat my dinner at around 7:30 p.m. Then I have a little something like a banana, a bowl of berries with chocolate chips, or some cucumbers and hummus at around 9:30 p.m., just before I go to bed. I did this when I was on my journey to lose seventy pounds, and in no way did it slow me down. You could also have a snack at around 5:00 p.m. and then eat dinner later in the evening. This is especially helpful to anyone who struggles with nighttime binging.

3. **Find lower-calorie swaps.** When you think about the foods you love and find lower-calorie alternatives, you'll be amazed by how much easier it is to cut calories while still feeling like you can eat food that makes you happy. Which is huge! It's also an easy way to shave off the extra calories that are lurking in your diet and keeping you from losing more weight. Here are some of my favorite low-calorie products:

IF YOU LOVE . . .	TRY . . .
Pasta	konjac noodles, kelp noodles, zucchini noodles, spaghetti squash
Bread	rice cakes, Ezekiel 4:9 sprouted bread (I love this bread because it's whole-grain, oil-free, and low in sodium. The sprouting of the grains also decreases the amount of gluten in the bread, which is great for those who are gluten sensitive or who are watching their gluten intake.)
Pizza crust	Low-calorie pita such as Joseph's 60-calorie pitas
Tortillas	Ole Extreme Wellness 50-calorie tortillas, Joseph's low-calorie wraps and 60-calorie pitas
Crackers	Edward and Sons oil-free rice crackers
Maple syrup	Lakanto all-natural sugar-free maple syrup (Lakanto is sweetened with monk fruit, which is naturally sweet, low in calories, and lower on the glycemic index than maple syrup. It's a wonderful low-calorie way to enjoy the flavor of syrup with your breakfast!)
Sweeteners	Monkfruit or liquid stevia. I love the flavored stevia by Now Brand Foods (toffee and French vanilla are out of this world)!
Soda and cocktails	All-natural sugar-free soft drinks such as the ones by Zevia that are sweetened with stevia; make your own "mocktails" by adding a splash of juice or fresh pureed fruit to all-natural flavored sparkling water.
Pasta sauce	Look for low-fat and oil-free marinara. I like the Whole Foods 365 brand.

CHAPTER 4

Plan for Success

A s the saying goes, "When you fail to plan, you plan to fail." In my experience, this couldn't be more true, especially when it comes to setting a weight-loss goal.

There's never as much time or energy as you think there's going to be when it comes to making a meal, and deciding what to eat when you feel rushed or are already ravenous can derail even the best-intentioned among us. That's why being prepared with the right equipment in your kitchen, the right snacks on hand, the right meals prepped ahead of time, and the right know-how for navigating a restaurant menu is what will ultimately help you finish strong. Because we've all been there—tired and hungry, reaching for foods that aren't in line with what we know is good for us. In this chapter, we'll talk about other ways you can support yourself and set yourself up for success, such as moving consistently throughout the day and, most important, doing things that bring you joy and make you feel good. The more you find genuine connection and pleasure in it, the better your results will be!

Prep Your Meals

Meal prep is absolutely essential to your success. Consider it this way: You need to eat at least three times a day—ideally more, if you include snacks—every single day. And bringing your life to a halt each and every time to first decide what you'd like to eat and then prepare it isn't just unrealistic, it's detrimental to your success. Because what will inevitably happen in those moments of urgency or hunger is that you'll reach for food that isn't aligned with your goals. And doing that over and over again, even if it's not every day, is like death by a thousand cuts.

Take a little time every week to plan what you'd like to eat and prep accordingly—and I really do mean a little. (See Meal Prep in Five Easy Steps on the next page.) You can do this any time of day and any day of the week. Some people assume this all has to happen on Sunday afternoons, but those can sometimes be the busiest days. Figure out what works for you, then pencil it in and stick to it like you would an appointment. Even if it's only twenty minutes, see what you can get done during that time; I guarantee it'll be more than you think, and it'll buy you so much more time during the week, not to mention set you up for making the best meal and snack choices possible. During my prep time, I like to

- cook my starches (rice, pasta, potatoes)
- mix up a couple of dressings
- chop any veggies I might want to toss into a salad (buying pre-chopped veggies is also a great idea)

Everything can be stored in airtight containers in the fridge and will last all week, meaning a satisfying meal with ingredients I want to eat is never more than a few minutes away. It's also a good idea to keep a stash of

Meal Prep in Five Easy Steps

Choose your meals for the week. I make double batches of three main dishes and then rotate them for lunch and dinner Sunday through Thursday. I plan for one or two meals that I want to enjoy on the weekend. See pages 47–56 for meal plans or pages 69–244 for all the recipes.

Select your snacks, including lots of fresh fruit and vegetables.

Wash, chop, and store your produce.

Prep your starches (potatoes, rice, pasta).

Make your sauces and condiments. Choose one thing for dipping, something spicy, and something you can use as both a marinade and a sauce. (See Chapter 9 for all my favorite recipes.)

frozen veggies in the freezer, which are great for quickly steaming.

My recipes typically make enough for one serving because individuals following this eating plan tend to be cooking for themselves and would prefer not to have a bunch of leftovers. However, the recipes can be scaled up for additional servings, whether it's because you want to batch cook the components, have more leftovers for later in the week, or serve others. Many of these recipes are favorites in my family!

Here's what you should aim to prep for the week to make pulling meals together easier:

Prep Your Snacks

It's also imperative to have healthy snacks handy. It's way too easy to mindlessly graze on crackers or chips, or to get so hungry that you devour whatever's within arm's reach for your next meal, thereby taking in far more calories than you intended to. Instead, keep a stash of fruits and veggies with low calorie density. If you need something more filling, see Chapter 9 for great healthy dip recipes that you can enjoy along with a low-calorie pita (see Food Products I Love). Just make sure you remember to track your caloric intake—yes, snacks count too!

Prep Your Kitchen

You'll have a much easier time making goal-friendly meals if you have the right kitchen equipment and ingredients. With some smart staples, you'll not only feel prepared to take on a week's worth of delicious dishes but you'll also be able to whip something up at a moment's notice, if necessary. Here are some of my favorites.

HELPFUL KITCHEN TOOLS

High-speed blender, such as Vitamix or Blendtec

Small high-speed blender, such as NutriBullet or Ninja (for making smaller amounts of dressings and condiments)

Digital kitchen scale

A good chef's knife

Microplane grater

Air fryer

Rice cooker

Medium and large nonstick pots and pans

Instant Pot or other multicooker

FOOD PRODUCTS I LOVE

Bouillon cubes: Edward and Sons Not Chick'n Bouillon Cubes

Bread: Ezekiel 4:9 bread

Chocolate chips: Enjoy Life and Lakanto chocolate chips

Cooking spray: Chosen Foods avocado oil cooking spray

Crackers: Edward and Sons oil-free rice crackers

Hot sauce: Sambal oelek

Maple syrup (sugar free): Lakanto all-natural sugar-free maple syrup

Pasta sauce: 365 brand fat-free marinara

Peanut butter: PB2 powdered peanut butter

Pita: Joseph's low-calorie lavash and pita

Sweetener: Monk fruit or liquid stevia, especially the flavored stevia by Now Brand Foods (toffee and French vanilla are my favorites)

Tortillas: Ole Extreme Wellness 50-calorie Tortillas

Whipped cream: Reddi-Wip almond milk whipped cream

Yogurt: So Delicious coconut yogurt

Prep for Eating Out

Eating in a restaurant can create anxiety for people who are following a low-calorie diet, but it can be easier to navigate than you'd think. I always start by reviewing the menu online whenever possible. If I don't see something I can eat, I'll call the restaurant ahead of time and ask if the kitchen can prepare any of the following:

- A salad with vinaigrette on the side
- Steamed veggies and steamed rice with teriyaki sauce on the side
- Fresh rice-paper rolls with veggie filling and rice noodles with a side of dipping sauce
- Steamed vegetable dumplings
- Vegetable soups (cream-free)
- Steamed or baked potato with ketchup or steak sauce on the side
- Vegetable pizza without cheese (think of it as a veggie flatbread)

- Burrito bowl with rice, beans, salsa, lettuce, and guacamole
- Bean enchiladas with lettuce, guacamole, salsa, and enchilada sauce
- Coconut vegetable curry
- Chickpea curry and rice
- Vegetable and hummus sandwich

Restaurants across North America are expanding their menus to include plant-based options, so it's usually easy to find something to eat. Still, I often preload with a filling salad or a bowl of soup (see page 190). That's it! Now you're free to enjoy your evening.

The more prepared you are and the clearer your plan, the more successful you'll be. Winging it never goes as well as expected. It almost always leads to eating foods you wouldn't normally choose to have, and often eating more of them.

Take a Break from Alcohol

I strongly recommend cutting back on alcohol, if not eliminating it altogether—for now. It's just way too easy to overconsume these liquid calories; plus, even a little buzz can stir your cravings for high-calorie foods or cause you to eat more food than you normally would. A Danish study published in 2002 in the *International Journal of Obesity and Related Metabolic Disorders* found that people ate more when their meal was served with beer or wine instead of soda.

Also, consider the physiological effects alcohol has on your body. Your liver sees alcohol as a toxin, so in order to deal with this intruding substance, it slows down its fat-burning function (one of its many important roles), sometimes for up to forty-eight hours after you've had a drink. On top of that, alcohol will cause you to retain water for the next day or two as your body attempts to rehydrate itself.

Instead of choosing alcoholic beverages to sip socially or accompany your meals, I suggest having fun with natural sugar-free drinks such as Zevia, which is sweetened with stevia. (Stevia is derived from the leaf of the stevia plant—a relative of the sunflower—which has been used in Asia for decades as a table sweetener and is one of my favorite ways to add sweetness to my own recipes.)

A great mocktail is just as satisfying as a cocktail, in my opinion, and with a fraction of the calories. You can get as creative as you want with flavored stevia drops. One of my favorite creations is the Mock Coconut Mojito: Mix together sparkling water, a few drops of coconut-flavored stevia, lime juice, and a small handful of fresh mint leaves. Or add lime, cucumber, or fresh berries to your water for tasty "spa" water.

Aim for Daily Activity

Daily activity is not only key to maintaining a calorie deficit, it's also important for your overall health. But that doesn't mean you need to spend hours at the gym or get hard-core with CrossFit—unless, of course, that sounds like fun to you. (It doesn't to me!) Instead, think of exercise the way you do your food—it should be something you enjoy, or these lifestyle shifts won't be sustainable.

I had an important exercise breakthrough when I finally came to terms with the fact that I hate high-intensity exercise in all its forms. Once I made peace with that and gave myself permission to look for another kind of exercise that genuinely brought me joy, my entire relationship with exercise changed. I began walking every day. Exercise suddenly no longer felt like a chore or, worse, something I dreaded. Instead, the opposite happened; it lit a spark in me. Now I have gear for any kind of weather—rain, shine, wind, or snow—so I don't have to skip a day, and because I love being out in nature, I'm always looking for new trails to explore or mountains to climb. If my family or a friend wants to join, even better! The genuine enjoyment I got out of walking and hiking meant that I did it more, and the more I did it, the more ingrained it became in my life. And the best part of all is that I didn't do anything more intense than walking during my entire weight-loss journey.

So, the first important step when it comes to exercise is to find something you love without getting too caught up with the "shoulds." The second piece is committing to move your body for thirty to forty minutes every day. When I was first starting out with my exercise routine,

I set this goal for myself and then enlisted my friend Nicole to be my accountability buddy. Every day we texted each other—complete with a selfie—to say that we'd hit our goal. Some days I could do it all at once, but other days I had to break it into three or four ten-minute walks—and that's okay! Over time, in addition to adding some weight-lifting workouts such as simple squats, lunges, and shoulder exercises with free weights into the mix, I've worked up to longer stretches of daily activity. I've committed to ten thousand steps a day, which takes about an hour to an hour and ten minutes of brisk walking. But, if need be, I still break it up into several shorter walks so I can hit my goal no matter what my schedule looks like. And to this day, my bestie and I send each other pics of our steps!

Don't feel like you need to get to an hour right out of the gate. In fact, don't feel pressure to hit the hour mark at all. Start with thirty to forty minutes and see how you feel. And if you can, put a buddy system in place so that you don't feel like you're in this alone. I'm willing to bet there's someone in your life who wants to root you on, and your experience will be that much more consistent and fulfilling for it.

Get Your Steps, Steps, and More Steps!

Walking is one of the easiest ways to hit your movement goal and create a consistent caloric deficit, no matter what your preferred primary form of exercise is. You can stroll with your thoughts (or music or a podcast), stroll with a friend, stroll with your family, stroll on your way to do errands, stroll in nature, stroll

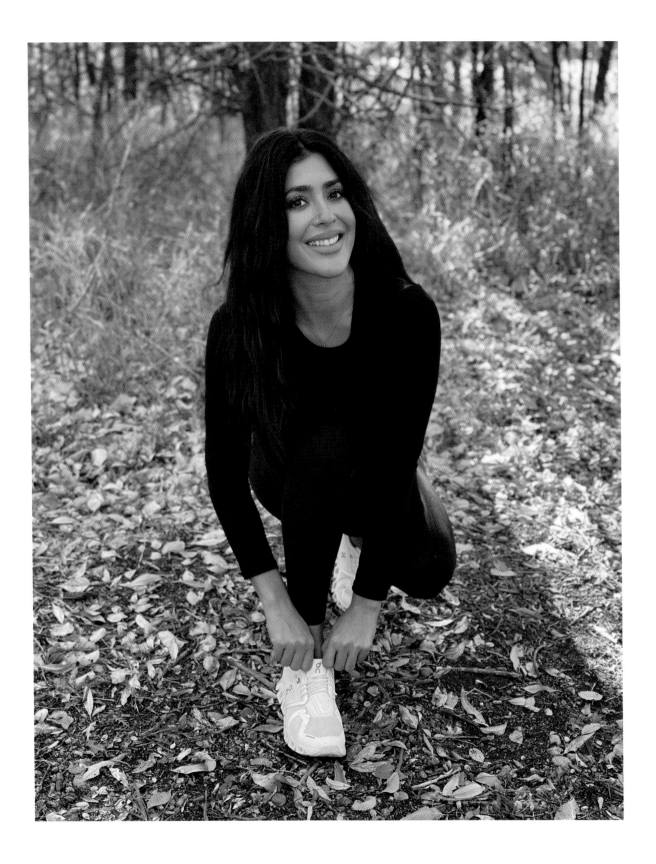

in the city, stroll anywhere, anytime! It may not always feel like you're doing much, but your body reaps major benefits from all that consistent, prolonged, gentle movement.

It has the ability to:

- Boost circulation
- Stabilize your blood sugar
- Increase your energy levels throughout the day
- Reduce muscle stiffness and joint pain
- Reduce high blood pressure and the risk of heart disease and stroke
- Improve digestive health
- Improve your sleep
- Improve your mood
- Pretty much improve your life all around

Consider this: According to Dan Buettner, the founder of Blue Zones and an expert on the healthiest populations around the world, the people on this planet with the longest life spans are those who average about twelve thousand steps a day (about five miles of walking).

Over time, I suggest working up to a goal of ten thousand steps a day. Yes, it's a lot, and it does take some mindful effort, but the upside is that it also happens to burn an average of four hundred calories. Begin with a smaller goal that feels realistic for you (I started with five thousand steps) and increase the number every week. I highly recommend that you invest in a step counter. Even if your phone has one, buy one that you wear, because it will be more accurate and you don't have to worry about always having your phone on you. (It can be nice to unplug, especially while getting in a much-

needed movement break.) If you already have an Apple Watch, you're good to go!

Ten Tips for Getting Those Steps In

1. Enlist a friend to join you either in person or in the same goal and send each other daily texts showing you completed your steps for the day. Make it fun!
2. Break up your workday with mini-walks—one in the morning, another at lunch, and a third after work.
3. Park at the back of the parking lot. All those errands start to add up!
4. Take the stairs instead of the elevator. (And give yourself a good reason to take multiple trips, like bringing up the laundry or groceries in batches.)
5. Instead of a coffee break, or after you've eaten lunch, take a brisk walking break. Invite a coworker to help pass the time and create built-in accountability—win-win!
6. Take a walking break during phone meetings and walk while you talk. The same goes for calls with your friends or family. It doesn't have to be outside; laps around your house count!
7. Consider investing in a walking desk (a desk attached to a treadmill). You'd be amazed how productive you can be while slowly walking on a treadmill—and how many steps you can get in over the course of the day.
8. If you take your kids to sports practice, walk laps around the field or court.
9. Make walks the new happy hour. It's the perfect way to catch up with friends while also getting in steps. Bonus points if you

pick up smoothies to sip on while you walk.

10. Get the family involved on the weekends. Choose new trails and parks for your adventures together.

Practice Self-Care

Committing to a healthy lifestyle and weight-loss journey will be challenging. All change is. But it need not be agonizing.

To make this process as fulfilling as it can be, lean into all the ways you can make it enjoyable. This begins with preparing foods and making sure that you're getting enough of the good stuff in your life, the things that make you feel your best, inside and out—for example, rest, mindfulness, gratitude, and joy. In order to do that, you need to take time for yourself.

This looks different for everyone, but it ultimately comes down to listening to what you need *and* what you want. If you feel tired, rest. If you're feeling energetic, spend that motivation on an activity that you enjoy. If you're feeling overwhelmed, reach for something that makes you feel calm. If you love reading, take time to sit somewhere peaceful and read. For me, it's knitting on my front porch or sitting at my breakfast table with some tea, markers, and an adult coloring book. Even my daughter and teenage son love to sit and color with me! Listen to that little voice inside you that's telling you what it needs and wants to feel nourished and happy.

Now, I know that for many of you, that might be just as challenging, if not more so, than making adjustments to your diet. I'm a mom; I get it.

Five Minutes to Bliss

- Take a short walk to recharge and reconnect with yourself. Play your favorite songs, recite your mantra (see page 40), or enjoy some peace and quiet. Remind yourself that you are amazing and worth taking care of.
- Spend time with your inspiration album. I keep a photo album on my phone (Pinterest is great for this) with images that remind me of what I'm working toward every day—places I want to visit with my family, home projects I'm excited to take on, flowers I want to plant in my garden, and so on. Just a few minutes of daydreaming about things that bring me joy is motivating and grounding.
- Take a music break. Whether it's uplifting and energizing or slow and soothing, choose a song to match your mood and spend that time softening into a new headspace.

The fact is, the more nourished and centered you are, the more you can show up for everyone around you. Luckily, just a few minutes here and there can often be enough to shift your entire vibration and help you feel a little more mellowed out or pumped up.

Perhaps the most important thing you can do for yourself is get at least seven to eight hours of sleep every night. This is one tenet of health that isn't controversial. Researchers agree that getting enough good, deep rest is key to optimal health, and that it's also essential for making better choices during the day. A tired brain is one that craves quick-hitting energy from high-sugar, high-fat sources, often processed foods. And those foods, in turn, make you lethargic. It's a vicious cycle. A few simple habits can make a big difference when it comes to getting more quality sleep:

Spend thirty minutes before bed winding down *without* a screen. (The blue light from electronic devices such as cell phones, laptops, and televisions can disrupt the production of melatonin, which is what helps you fall asleep.) I like journaling or reading a good romance novel (don't judge!) or a self-improvement book before dozing off.

Take the last five minutes before bed to reflect on the things you're grateful for in your life or just in your day. It will help clear your mind and make you feel grounded, which is the ideal state to be in to make drifting off to sleep easy.

Make your bedroom a dark, cool, and calm oasis. Any light (from windows or electronic devices) can disturb your melatonin production.

Your body naturally lowers its core temperature for sleep, so assisting with that process will make it easier to fall asleep and stay asleep. The more soothing an environment your bedroom is, the more relaxed you'll be. Add a sleep-promoting fragrance such as lavender, treat yourself to sheets that feel nice (they don't have to be expensive!), and remove any items that might be stressful to look at as you're lying in bed (work, laundry that needs to be folded, etc.).

The Mindset Miracle

Mindset is everything. If you're of the mindset that you can't eat healthy for your whole life, then you will certainly not eat healthy for your whole life. If you believe that you'll never be able to create new habits, then that will end up being your experience.

Your thoughts inform your feelings, your feelings inform your actions, and your actions create your experience. So, if you work on telling yourself that you love to take care of yourself and eat wholesome foods, then your actions will become an extension of your new beliefs, which will then become your reality.

Cultivating belief in yourself is crucial to your success. I encourage you to come up with a mantra or phrase that you carry with you. Ideally, it will be one that speaks to your specific challenges and strengthens your resolve. Here's what mine looked like years ago when I was first getting the hang of my new healthy habits:

I am healthy and beautiful. I show myself love by taking care of my body with good nutrition and plenty of sleep. I eat with intention because I deserve the effort and care it takes to be healthy. I love eating lots of fresh fruits and vegetables, and I love eating whole and minimally processed foods and fats. I find joy in my simple diet and comfort in knowing that I'm treating my body with love and respect. I am worthy, I am valuable, I am loved.

I kept this mantra taped to my place at our kitchen table so every time I sat down to eat, I was reminded of my new beliefs about myself, which helped me become the person I wanted to be. You could also write your mantra on a sticky note and leave it somewhere that you'll see it throughout the day, or write it in the food or activity journal you keep. Over time, you'll find that your mantra will become who you are at the core of your being. Remember, you deserve to feel good and take care of yourself. You are worth the time and effort that it takes. You are beautiful.

Putting It All Together

Below I've shared how I arrange my day to fit in the habits that make me feel rested, fueled, and happy. Not every day looks like this exactly, but I've set a high bar for myself because I know that if I carve out the time for each of these self-care elements, then there's a much greater chance I'll include them. And once I got into the rhythm of incorporating these practices, they became second nature.

Everyone's life looks different, of course, with various time constraints and obligations. And you may need to be selective about what you truly have time for. Or you may want to enlist some help to buy you a little more time in the day, such as swapping babysitting or dinner preparation duties with a friend. The key is to figure out what this can look like in your own life, and then get into a *consistent* routine. Even if at first you're dedicating only a few minutes to each new habit you want to build, the more consistent you are, the more ingrained these new habits will be, and the more effective the changes you'll make. If you want to change the results, you have to change the routine.

Here's an example of a day in my life:

5:30 A.M.: Wake up and drink a big glass of water.

5:40 A.M. TO 6:00 A.M.: Reflect on things I'm grateful for, go over my affirmations, and meditate in prayer.

6:00 A.M. TO 7:30 A.M.: Wake up the kids, have breakfast with them, and get them ready to catch the bus.

7:30 A.M. TO 8:00 A.M.: Thirty-minute walk outside with my dog.

8:00 A.M. TO 10:30 A.M.: Work, meetings, e-mail.

10:30 A.M. TO 10:45 A.M.: Snack (usually fruit or veggies and hummus) and ten-minute walk.

10:45 A.M. TO 1:00 P.M.: Work and meetings.

1:00 P.M. TO 1:30 P.M.: Lunch break.

1:30 P.M. TO 1:50 P.M.: Twenty-minute walk.

1:50 P.M. TO 2:50 P.M.: Work.

2:50 P.M. TO 3:10 P.M.: Twenty-minute walk to the bus stop to pick up the kids.

3:10 P.M. TO 3:50 P.M.: After-school snack with the kids (fruit or Joseph's pita with hummus)

3:50 P.M. TO 6:00 P.M.: Work.

6:00 P.M. TO 7:30 P.M.: Prepare dinner, eat with the family, family time, help with homework, kiss kids goodnight for their independent quiet time.

7:30 P.M. TO 8:30 P.M.: Cuddle on the couch with my husband and watch *Yellowstone*.

8:30 P.M. TO 9:00 P.M.: Shower or hot bath.

9:00 P.M. TO 9:30 P.M.: Read in bed.

9:30 P.M.: Lights out; I fall asleep giving thanks for all the blessings in my life.

Holding Yourself Accountable

You're setting exciting goals and envisioning a life where you show up for yourself in a significant way. While that's the necessary first step to creating change, continuing to make that change is where the real work happens. Repeat your new practices every day until they become ingrained habits and create a safety net for yourself in the form of accountability. These simple tools go a long way toward ensuring that you continue taking these important steps forward.

Identify your goals.

A good goal is one that's specific, achievable, and measurable. Simply saying "I will lose twenty pounds" is too open-ended and overwhelming. Instead, break it down into smaller pieces: "I will prep my meals for one week" or "I will hit five thousand steps for five days." If even those things seem daunting, keep narrowing down goals into bite-size pieces. Over time, these smaller goals add up to big achievements.

Write down your goals.

Nothing makes something feel more real than seeing it in writing. Record your goals where you can read them every morning and every evening.

Put them on the schedule. When people pencil in time for their meals, movement breaks, and self-care routine and then treat those things as they would a meeting or an appointment, they're much more likely to make good on those things. It also reinforces the very important—and very true—message that taking care of yourself is just as important as anything else you need to do that day.

Enlist an accountability partner. Not feeling like you're doing this alone—and not wanting to let your partner down—is a powerful motivator. Ask a friend, partner, family member, or coworker if they'd like to embark on this journey with you. Send each other pics of your meals and step counters throughout the day and share words of encouragement.

CHAPTER 5

28-Day Meal Plan: The Kickoff

To help you transition into this new approach to eating, I've created two different plans to help you meet your caloric needs while also introducing you to many of the great recipes in this book. Here's what's helpful to know:

If you're currently on Path 1 (page 21): These meal plans have you covered in the low-fat, plant-based diet department, so there's no need to do anything more than eat, enjoy, and listen to your biofeedback cues (or natural feeling of fullness). If these meal plans leave you feeling too hungry between meals, simply increase the amount you eat at meals or add snacks such as fresh fruit and veggies with one of the dips from Chapter 9. And while these recipes were created using my plate-building method (page 15), you can always begin your meals with additional nonstarchy vegetables.

If you're currently on Path 2 (page 22): Each day of both plans provides 1,200 to 2,000 calories, so you may need to make some adjustments given your specific requirements in order to maintain a 250- to 500-calorie deficit. For example, some of the dinner options are espe-cially low in calories, so it might be appropriate to double the serving size or add a dessert from Chapter 10.

For both paths: These plans are for meals only, so feel free to round things out with snacks. Remember, cutting back too sharply on calo-ries or not eating enough throughout the day is likely to lead to binging down the road. Be moderate in your approach and enjoy the deli-cious, healthy food that's available to you.

These plans are meant to be customized not only to your needs but also to your preferences. Never feel like you need to make a recipe simply because it's on the plan. Swap out any recipes that don't speak to you or repeat the ones that do.

Don't forget to prep! Getting a jump on mak-ing each week's meals will make this process so much easier and more enjoyable. See page 32 for a refresher on all my meal-prepping tips.

The Keep It Interesting 28-Day Meal Plan

This meal plan is for anyone who likes a lot of variety in their meals. So, if you easily get bored eating the same dish multiple times a week, this plan is for you. These recipes yield one or two servings, so you won't need to worry about generating too many leftovers or wasting food.

Week 1

	BREAKFAST	LUNCH	DINNER	TOTAL DAILY CALORIES
MONDAY	Chocolate Peanut Butter Smoothie (page 87) Calories: 468	Teriyaki Bowl (page 180) Calories: 548	Yellow Potato Curry (page 149) Calories: 516	1,532
TUESDAY	Blueberry Peach Crisp (page 79) Calories: 543	Yellow Potato Curry (page 149) Calories: 516	Food Truck Tacos (page 138) Calories: 352	1,411
WEDNESDAY	Garlic Herb Potato Waffles (page 102) Calories: 433	Food Truck Tacos (page 138) Calories: 352	Cauliflower Steak Dinner with Mashed Potatoes and Green Beans (page 150) Calories: 534	1,319
THURSDAY	Pineapple Ginger Smoothie (page 86) Calories: 436	Cauliflower Steak Dinner with Mashed Potatoes and Green Beans (page 150) Calories: 534	Mushroom Stroganoff (page 172) Calories: 450	1,420
FRIDAY	Lemon Berry Patch Yogurt (page 83) Calories: 389	Mushroom Stroganoff (page 172) Calories: 450	Spring Alfredo Pasta (page 166) Calories: 404	1,243
SATURDAY	Blueberry Lemon Oat Waffles (page 73) Calories: 459	Spring Alfredo Pasta (page 166) Calories: 404	Vegan Crab Cakes (page 154) Calories: 287	1,150
SUNDAY	Garden Vegetable Chickpea Omelet (page 98) Calories: 359	Vegan Crab Cakes (page 154) Calories: 287	Cheesy Poblano Enchiladas (page 161) Calories: 623	1,269

Week 2

	BREAKFAST	LUNCH	DINNER	TOTAL DAILY CALORIES
MONDAY	"Egg" and Avocado Breakfast Sandwich with 2 cups of grapes (page 106) Calories: 377	Cheesy Poblano Enchiladas (page 161) Calories: 623	Lentil Mushroom Stew (page 114) Calories: 384	1,384
TUESDAY	Coffee Caramel Smoothie (page 88) Calories: 502	Lentil Mushroom Stew (page 114) Calories: 384	Sesame Ginger Cold Noodle Bowl (page 183) Calories: 397	1,283
WEDNESDAY	Fruit Salsa with Cinnamon Toast (page 92) Calories: 438	Cilantro-Lime Stuffed Peppers (page 157) Calories: 563	Creamy Roasted Pepper Pasta (page 165) Calories: 540	1,541
THURSDAY	Raspberry Chocolate Muffins with 2 cups berries (page 71) Calories: 459	Cauliflower Steak Dinner with Mashed Potatoes and Green Beans (page 150) Calories: 534	Cilantro-Lime Stuffed Peppers (page 157) Calories: 563	1,556
FRIDAY	Mermaid Smoothie Bowl (page 91) Calories: 559	Creamy Roasted Pepper Pasta (page 165) Calories: 540	Saucy Portobello Sammies (page 129) Calories: 322	1,421
SATURDAY	Asian-Inspired Vegetable Pancakes (page 100) Calories: 472	Saucy Portobello Sammies (page 129) Calories: 322	Lean Lasagna (page 168) Calories: 627	1,421
SUNDAY	Raspberry Lemon Poppy Seed Pancakes (page 76) Calories: 360	Lean Lasagna (page 168) Calories: 627	Smoky Sweet Chili (page 174) Calories: 657	1,644

Week 3

	BREAKFAST	LUNCH	DINNER	TOTAL DAILY CALORIES
MONDAY	Coffee Caramel Smoothie (page 88) Calories: 502	Smoky Sweet Chili (page 174) Calories: 657	Japanese Nourish Bowl (page 186) Calories: 443	1,602
TUESDAY	Vanilla Berry Parfait with Chocolate Granola (page 69) Calories: 437	Japanese Nourish Bowl (page 186) Calories: 443	Hawaiian Potatoes (page 171) Calories: 634	1,514
WEDNESDAY	Blueberry Peach Crisp (page 79) Calories: 543	Hawaiian Potatoes (page 171) Calories: 634	Sweet Potato Black Bean Curry (page 109) Calories: 441	1,618
THURSDAY	Citrus Dragon Fruit Smoothie Bowl (page 89) Calories: 426	Sweet Potato Black Bean Curry (page 109) Calories: 441	Grilled "Steak" and Cheese Sammy x 2 (page 133) Calories: 536	1,403
FRIDAY	PB & J Smoothie Bowl (page 94) Calories: 533	Grilled "Steak" and Cheese Sammy x 2 (page 133) Calories: 536	Black Bean Tacos with Avocado Lime Crema (page 134) Calories: 427	1,496
SATURDAY	Chocolate Peanut Butter Oatmeal (page 84) Calories: 455	Black Bean Tacos with Avocado Lime Crema (page 134) Calories: 427	Lean Lasagna (page 168) Calories: 627	1,509
SUNDAY	Mushroom Steak and "Eggs" with Herby Caesar (page 97) Calories: 367	Fajita Bowl (page 184) Calories: 562	Mexican Hash Brown Bake (page 158) Calories: 551	1,480

Week 4

	BREAKFAST	LUNCH	DINNER	TOTAL DAILY CALORIES
MONDAY	"Egg" and Avocado Breakfast Sandwich with 2 oranges, sliced (page 106) Calories: 377	Mexican Hash Brown Bake (page 184) Calories: 551	Sloppy Joe Pockets (page 127) Calories: 651	1,579
TUESDAY	Raspberry Chocolate Muffins with 2 cups of berries (page 71) Calories: 459	Sloppy Joe Pockets (page 127) Calories: 651	Pesto Pasta Primavera (page 162) Calories: 470	1,580
WEDNESDAY	Chocolate Peanut Butter Smoothie (page 87) Calories: 468	Pesto Pasta Primavera (page 162) Calories: 470	Loaded Taco Sweet Potato (page 142) Calories: 529	1,467
THURSDAY	Lemon Berry Patch Yogurt (page 83) Calories: 389	Loaded Taco Sweet Potato (page 142) Calories: 529	Peanut Soba Noodles (page 177) Calories: 513	1,431
FRIDAY	Coffee Caramel Smoothie (page 88) Calories: 502	Peanut Soba Noodles (page 177) Calories: 513	Hawaiian Street Cart Tacos (page 137) Calories: 372	1,387
SATURDAY	Asian-Inspired Vegetable Pancakes (page 100) Calories: 472	Hawaiian Street Cart Tacos (page 137) Calories: 372	Cauliflower Steak Dinner with Mashed Potatoes and Green Beans (page 150) Calories: 534	1,378
SUNDAY	Blueberry Lemon Oat Waffles (page 73) Calories: 459	Cauliflower Steak Dinner with Mashed Potatoes and Green Beans (page 150) Calories: 534	Smoky Sweet Chili (page 174) Calories: 657	1,650

———

The best way to eat a low-fat,
plant-based diet consistently
is to make sure that you always
have the option of eating
something you truly enjoy.

———

The Keep It Simple 28-Day Meal Plan

For every person who won't even look at leftovers, there's someone who loves nothing more than repetition in their meals. I happen to like repeating the recipes I'm making for the week because it streamlines the grocery shopping and prep. This is a great plan if you're newer to cooking your own meals or you're short on time.

Week 1

	BREAKFAST	LUNCH	DINNER	TOTAL DAILY CALORIES
MONDAY	Chocolate Peanut Butter Smoothie (page 87) Calories: 468	Smoky Sweet Chili (page 174) Calories: 657	Teriyaki Bowl (page 180) Calories: 548	1,673
TUESDAY	Coffee Caramel Smoothie (page 88) Calories: 502	Smoky Sweet Chili (page 174) Calories: 657	Teriyaki Bowl (page 180) Calories: 548	1,707
WEDNESDAY	Vanilla Berry Parfait with Chocolate Granola (page 69) Calories: 437	Falafel Cauliflower Pitas (page 120) Calories: 405	Mushroom Stroganoff (page 172) Calories: 450	1,292
THURSDAY	Vanilla Berry Parfait with Chocolate Granola (page 69) Calories: 437	Falafel Cauliflower Pitas (page 120) Calories: 405	Mushroom Stroganoff (page 172) Calories: 450	1,292
FRIDAY	Blueberry Peach Crisp (page 79) Calories: 543	Herby White Bean Sammy (page 124) Calories: 465	Hawaiian Street Cart Tacos (page 137) Calories: 372	1,380
SATURDAY	Garden Vegetable Chickpea Omelet (page 98) Calories: 359	Herby White Bean Sammy (page 124) Calories: 465	Veggie Supreme Pita Pizzas (page 146) Calories: 360	1,184
SUNDAY	Mushroom Steak and "Eggs" with Herby Caesar (page 97) Calories: 367	Hawaiian Potatoes (page 171) Calories: 634	Sweet Potato Black Bean Curry (page 109) Calories: 623	1,624

Week 2

	BREAKFAST	LUNCH	DINNER	TOTAL DAILY CALORIES
MONDAY	Mushroom Steak and "Eggs" with Herby Caesar (page 97) Calories: 367	Hawaiian Potatoes (page 171) Calories: 634	Sweet Potato Black Bean Curry (page 109) Calories: 623	1,624
TUESDAY	"Egg" and Avocado Breakfast Sandwich (page 106) Calories: 377	Everything Bagel Wrap (page 118) Calories: 444	Japanese Nourish Bowl (page 186) Calories: 443	1,264
WEDNESDAY	"Egg" and Avocado Breakfast Sandwich (page 106) Calories: 377	Everything Bagel Wrap (page 118) Calories: 444	Japanese Nourish Bowl (page 186) Calories: 443	1,264
THURSDAY	Blueberry Peach Crisp (page 79) Calories: 543	Peanut Soba Noodles (page 177) Calories: 513	Food Truck Tacos (page 138) Calories: 352	1,408
FRIDAY	Blueberry Peach Crisp (page 79) Calories: 543	Peanut Soba Noodles (page 177) Calories: 513	Food Truck Tacos (page 138) Calories: 352	1,408
SATURDAY	Raspberry Lemon Poppy Seed Pancakes (page 76) Calories: 360	Sweet Potato Black Bean Curry (page 109) Calories: 623	Hawaiian Potatoes (page 171) Calories: 634	1,617
SUNDAY	Raspberry Lemon Poppy Seed Pancakes (page 76) Calories: 360	Loaded Taco Sweet Potato (page 142) Calories: 529	Lentil Mushroom Stew (page 114) Calories: 384	1,273

Week 3

	BREAKFAST	LUNCH	DINNER	TOTAL DAILY CALORIES
MONDAY	Garden Vegetable Chickpea Omelet (page 98) Calories: 359	Loaded Taco Sweet Potato (page 142) Calories: 529	Lentil Mushroom Stew (page 114) Calories: 384	1,272
TUESDAY	Garden Vegetable Chickpea Omelet (page 98) Calories: 359	Creamy Roasted Pepper Pasta (page 165) Calories: 540	Saucy Portobello Sammies (page 129) Calories: 322	1,221
WEDNESDAY	Pineapple Ginger Smoothie (page 86) Calories: 436	Creamy Roasted Pepper Pasta (page 165) Calories: 540	Saucy Portobello Sammies (page 129) Calories: 322	1,298
THURSDAY	PB & J Smoothie Bowl (page 94) Calories: 533	Cilantro-Lime Stuffed Peppers (page 157) Calories: 563	Vegan Crab Cakes (page 154) Calories: 287	1,383
FRIDAY	Blueberry Peach Crisp (page 79) Calories: 543	Cilantro-Lime Stuffed Peppers (page 157) Calories: 563	Vegan Crab Cakes (page 154) Calories: 287	1,393
SATURDAY	Blueberry Peach Crisp (page 79) Calories: 543	Fajita Bowl (page 184) Calories: 562	Cauliflower Masala (page 153) Calories: 614	1,719
SUNDAY	Gardener's Breakfast (page 105) Calories: 297	Fajita Bowl (page 184) Calories: 562	Cauliflower Masala (page 153) Calories: 614	1,473

Week 4

	BREAKFAST	LUNCH	DINNER	TOTAL DAILY CALORIES
MONDAY	Gardener's Breakfast (page 105) Calories: 297	Apple Pimento Grilled Cheese with Caramelized Onions and Arugula (page 125) Calories: 474	Jackfruit Enchilada Tacos (page 141) Calories: 679	1,450
TUESDAY	"Egg" and Avocado Breakfast Sandwich (page 106) Calories: 377	Apple Pimento Grilled Cheese with Caramelized Onions and Arugula (page 125) Calories: 474	Jackfruit Enchilada Tacos (page 141) Calories: 679	1,530
WEDNESDAY	"Egg" and Avocado Breakfast Sandwich (page 106) Calories: 377	Sloppy Joe Pockets (page 127) Calories: 651	Mexican Hash Brown Bake (page 184) Calories: 551	1,579
THURSDAY	Vanilla Berry Parfait with Chocolate Granola (page 69) Calories: 437	Sloppy Joe Pockets (page 127) Calories: 651	Mexican Hash Brown Bake (page 184) Calories: 551	1,639
FRIDAY	Vanilla Berry Parfait with Chocolate Granola (page 69) Calories: 437	Teriyaki Bowl (page 180) Calories: 548	Black Bean Tacos with Avocado Lime Crema (page 134) Calories: 427	1,412
SATURDAY	Raspberry Lemon Poppy Seed Pancakes (page 76) Calories: 360	Teriyaki Bowl (page 180) Calories: 548	Black Bean Tacos with Avocado Lime Crema (page 134) Calories: 427	1,335
SUNDAY	Raspberry Lemon Poppy Seed Pancakes (page 76) Calories: 360	Smoky Sweet Chili (page 174) Calories: 657	Veggie Supreme Pita Pizzas (page 146) Calories: 360	1,377

Because both calorie-counting and non-calorie-counting approaches to losing weight are highly effective and appropriate for all individuals, you just need to pick what feels right—or, more important, what feels enjoyable and satisfying.

CHAPTER 6

Healthy Ever After: The Maintenance Path

I f you've gotten to this chapter, then the amazing news is that you've finally reached a weight that feels right to you and that you now want to maintain. That said, I also know *very* well how it can be just as daunting to maintain your new weight as it was to get there in the first place.

Maintenance often comes with the anxiety of wondering whether you'll be able to preserve the health marker or weight loss results you've worked so hard to achieve. But if you've followed either of my methods for steady weight loss without too extreme a calorie deficit and plenty of hearty, filling meals you love, then you already know how to make a low-fat, plant-based diet work for you. This is different from losing weight on a crash diet only for the results to come undone when you go back to "eating normally."

The *Plantifully Simple* approach sets you up for a lifetime of success because it's a lifestyle that delivers the home run of keeping you satisfied at mealtimes, improving your overall health, and, as a result, making you feel about your new health and weight. There is no return to "normal"—this *is* the new normal!

This is not to say that you can't ever enjoy the foods you used to love; I am, after all, all about balance. But you might find that, like me, you don't love the way you feel after eating these foods and that it's ultimately not worth it.

I enjoy the occasional less healthy restaurant meal from time to time, along with store-bought vegan cheese and crackers or a vegan maple doughnut from Whole Foods. But most of the time, I don't really feel the need. That's partially because my tastes have changed and I now crave the delicious meals that I'm making every day and also because I can truly feel the difference between eating low-fat, plant-based foods and those that contain more additives.

Ultimately, this phase of your journey has a little more flexibility, because you don't need to be as aware of maintaining a calorie deficit. You've already mastered the principles of calorie density, plate building, calorie deficit, and moderation. You've developed the daily habits to keep yourself on track. But there are also some tips and pointers I'd like to share that are specific to this phase, so let's break it down further.

How to Know You're Ready to Move to the Maintenance Path

One great way to know is if you've hit your health and weight-loss goals. Another is if you no longer want to continue your calorie deficit or want to take a temporary break from your weight-loss path.

It might sound surprising, but transitioning to the maintenance path before you hit your previously set weight-loss goal can be a useful tool for continuing to make healthy choices. Many individuals who've been in a calorie deficit for a month or two want to take a few weeks off. They don't want to derail their progress, just hit the pause button. Maintenance breaks can also come in handy when you have upcoming events or travel and you want the peace of mind that comes with knowing you'll be able to build healthy meals without as much structure and planning. The holidays are another great time to maintain. All of this is to say that the maintenance path is here for you whenever you need or want it!

Changing Gears

Eating low-fat, plant-based foods to your natural satiation point is a recipe for encouraging your body to settle at its ideal weight, so shifting to the maintenance path won't look much different for those of you on Path 1. Continue being mindful of the foods you're eating and how you're eating them (i.e., the balanced plate), and continue monitoring your hunger cues and biofeedback. If you're hungry, add more food. If you're not, let it ride. You can also try adding more higher-fat plant foods such as avocado and nuts and see how your body responds. It's as easy as that!

For those on Path 2, while maintaining your ideal weight does require the same mindfulness as losing weight, there's a little more wiggle room. During the weight-loss phase, you're focused on creating a consistent calorie deficit to engender weight loss. To maintain the weight you're currently at, however, you no longer need that deficit. That means you can eat more calories: Some people like to eat larger portions or add avocado to their meals, while others go for snacks and desserts or having a meal out every so often. The only guideline you'll be following—

aside from continuing to choose low-fat, plant-based foods—is to not exceed your daily caloric limit.

When beginning the maintenance path, the first thing you need to do is calculate the daily caloric limit that's going to put you into energy balance—meaning you're taking in the exact number of calories that your body is expending. You can do this either by using the TDEE calculator on page 22 or by multiplying your current weight by fifteen. For example, if you currently weigh 135 pounds and multiply that by fifteen, you get 2,025, which is your new caloric limit for maintaining your weight.

Now that you know how many calories you have to play with every day, I do want to revisit the idea that all you need to do is choose how you want to use them. Remember that junk food can be a slippery slope and can lead to reestablishing old habits that no longer serve you, and to exceeding your daily calorie target. Build the majority of your diet around the foods that you've been eating on your journey until this point, then use the leftover calories to sprinkle in things like extra servings, another drizzle of sauce or dressing, snacks, a second helping of a dessert from Chapter 10, or the occasional night out or treat.

If you continue with the habits you've created, then you'll be successful.

Tips for Long-Term Success

Preparation and consistency are the two major keys to beating weight regain.

Calculate your maintenance calories (if following Path 2). See page 24 to refresh your memory on how not to succumb to calorie goal–calculating pitfalls.

Plan your meals for the week, down to the snacks and desserts you want to add in with your new calorie limit. I've included a What I Eat in a Week section on page 62, which you can use for reference. Or you can refer to the meal plan in Chapter 5, keeping in mind that you will likely need to adjust slightly to accommodate your higher daily caloric goal.

Use the recipes in Part II for inspiration and to keep things varied and interesting. You won't get bored if you mix up what you eat. You can also check out the recipes in my first book, *Plantifully Lean*, or the recipes I'm always posting on my website and social media platforms.

Prep, prep, prep! Weekly meal prep is a must. Those who take the time to prep their meals so that they can stay on track even during busy days maintain their weight because they're setting themselves up for success. See page 32 for all my favorite meal prep tips. If all else fails and you can only prep one thing, make it your sauces, because they give flavor to all your dishes. If you have time for one more thing, make it your starches, which take longer to cook than nonstarchy vegetables and so are more difficult to throw together on the fly.

Don't forget about calorie density. Remember that the foods lowest in calorie density are going to be the highest in nutrition and bulk, meaning you can eat more of them and feel fuller without putting a big dent in your daily calories. Building meals around these foods will ensure your success. See page 29 for a handy list of them, as well as simple swaps.

Continue tracking calories (if on Path 1). At least for a little while, especially if you're someone who knows the regain game well. If you want to be absolutely sure you won't gain the weight back, then track calories until you feel confident in your routine and how you're building meals. I've found that simply sticking with low-fat, plant-based foods is enough to know that my weight isn't going to budge; counting calories is one tool available to you, but certainly not a required one for a lifetime of weight-loss success.

Keep a daily food and activity journal. This isn't just an effective practice for losing weight; it can also keep you on track in the maintenance phase. I encourage all my clients to do this, and to not only write down what they ate or the exercise they performed but also record their thoughts and feelings surrounding their choices. It's a powerful reminder of why you're making these decisions and of all the hard work that went into your feeling as good as you do now.

Be consistent. Notice that I didn't say perfect! Perfect doesn't exist—so don't hold yourself to that expectation. Your food choices may not always be what you'd hoped they would, or your weight may even go up, but as Dori says, "Just keep swimming." Come back to your tools and habits, be consistent, and you *will* get there.

Keep a clean environment. Dr. Douglas J. Lisle, author of *The Pleasure Trap*, says that one of the best ways to keep from eating junk food is to keep it out of your house. He refers to this as "keeping a clean environment."[1] This sounds simple, and it's very effective—especially if you struggle with staying away from junk food. Instead, fill your kitchen with loads of fresh, colorful fruits and vegetables that you can eat as is or dip in the different dressings and dips I've shared in this book. If it's not possible for you to keep a clean environment at work, the next best thing is bringing your food with you and having it available to snack on throughout the day. Think of it as taking the extra step to make yourself feel special and taken care of. You deserve to eat foods that will increase your well-being!

What I Eat in a Week

To give you an idea of what maintenance mode can look like meals-wise, I want to show you what I eat over the course of a week. Keep in mind that I've customized this plan to suit my body and activity level, so if it speaks to you, use it as a guide—but if it doesn't, use one of the other plans on pages 47–50 or 53–56. Most important, you'll see that I enjoy dessert, snacks, and more avocado and nut dressings than I would if I were in weight-loss mode.

Ultimately, being in maintenance mode means eating more of the foods you love, which for me are avocados, cheese sauce, and dressings. If the meals on the next page seem like too

much cooking or variety, then simplify things by doubling or even tripling your recipes in order to have leftovers for the next few nights or to pack up as lunch.

Meal prep is key for me, because it streamlines my cooking. There's nothing wrong with eating the same things over and over again for weeks on end! In the beginning of my journey, I relied on baked potatoes and cheese sauce and spaghetti for what seemed like months and still managed to get the vitamins and nutrients I needed. They were easy to prepare, and they sounded tasty to me at the time—win-win.

Your plan needs to be sustainable for you. Don't make your life more complicated than it needs to be!

The Art of Readjusting

After all the time you spent losing weight and the laser-like focus it required—which for many people is over the course of months or even years—it can feel a little strange to finally be able to say "I made it." And because of that, it can be even more disheartening if you see the number on the scale start moving in the wrong direction again. That's why I like to tell people that they need to master the art of readjusting—meaning they need to get used to the fact that life happens and sometimes we need to adjust.

I hear this all the time: "I was doing so well, but then I had to have surgery/went on vacation/have been busy with work, and I gained weight." Oftentimes these people feel like they're starting

---

1   Douglas J. Lisle, PhD, and Alan Goldhamer, DC, *The Pleasure Trap: Mastering the Force That Undermines Health & Happiness* (Healthy Living Publications, 2006).

	MONDAY	TUESDAY	WEDNESDAY	THURSDAY	FRIDAY	SATURDAY	SUNDAY
BREAKFAST	Pineapple Ginger Smoothie (page 86)	Breakfast Salad (page 80)	Blueberry Peach Crisp (page 79)	PB & J Smoothie Bowl (page 94)	Garden Vegetable Chickpea Omelet (page 98)	Mushroom Steak and "Eggs" with Herby Caesar (page 97)	Gardener's Breakfast (page 105)
SNACK	Grapes	Apple Slices	Pears	Peaches	Grapes	Pineapple	Banana
LUNCH	Samosa Wraps (page 123)	Smoky Sweet Chili (page 174)	Loaded Taco Sweet Potato (page 142)	Japanese Nourish Bowl (page 186)	Japanese Nourish Bowl (page 186)	Apple Pimento Grilled Cheese with Caramelized Onions and Arugula (page 125)	Saucy Portobello Sammies (page 129)
SNACK	Joseph's Pita and Simple Hummus (page 202)	Cucumber Slices and Mango Salsa (page 209)	Red Pepper Slices and Summer Guac (page 210)	Everything Bagel Bean Dip and Cucumber Slices (page 205)	Rice Crackers and Pico de Gallo (page 208)	Pita and Herby Bean Dip (page 206)	Lettuce Wraps with Mango Salsa (page 209)
DINNER	Smoky Sweet Chili (page 174)	Cauliflower Steak Dinner with Mashed Potatoes and Green Beans (page 150)	Japanese Nourish Bowl (page 186)	Black Bean Tacos with Avocado Lime Crema (page 134)	Veggie Supreme Pita Pizzas (page 146)	Sesame Ginger Cold Noodle Bowl (page 183)	Mexican Hash Brown Bake (page 184)
DESSERT	Peaches and Cream (page 234)	Apple Turnovers (page 238)	Cherry Pie Bowl (page 241)	Vanilla Tapioca Pudding (page 227)	Coffee-Chocolate Nice Cream (page 235)	Strawberry Shortcake (page 232)	One-Bowl Heavenly Banana Brownies (page 228)

all over again. But they're *not* starting over. And they're definitely not failures.

If there's one thing that's to be expected in life, it's the unexpected. All you need to do is readjust, refocus, and continue keeping an eye on your goals. Employ the tools you've honed over the course of this process and keep going. I readjust all the time! Especially after a vacation or a holiday break, I'm constantly going back to the basics. These resources will always be there for you, but you also have to be there for yourself, which brings me to the next topic: mindset.

Maintain a Self-Care Routine

Making yourself a priority isn't only important when you're actively trying to lose weight; it's the basis for a happy, healthy life. I always say, "What we feed our souls is just as important as what we feed our bodies." Now that you're in maintenance mode, self-care should be a well-established part of a new daily routine that includes:

- Seven to nine hours of sleep
- Proper nutrition (i.e., food that gives you nourishment, pleasure, and vitality)
- Thirty to forty minutes of daily movement you enjoy
- At least one moment of rest and relaxation a day (such as reading, journaling, meditating, or deep breathing; see Five Minutes to Bliss on page 39)

If at first it seems challenging to establish a routine, focus on tackling one area at a time—maybe sleep or taking a brisk morning walk. Then, once you have one habit down, move on to the next. All the small changes you make will add up to big, lasting change. Keep working on these new habits until you have a daily routine that you can stick with and that brings you joy. See page 42 for what a day in my life looks like and how I like to sprinkle in all the self-care moments I can between parenting and work obligations. It's possible—especially if you continue to believe that you're worth it!

———

If at first it seems challenging to establish a routine, focus on tackling one area at a time—maybe sleep or taking a brisk morning walk. Then, once you have one habit down, move on to the next. All the small changes you make will add up to big, lasting change.

———

PART

2

Recipes for Delicious Meals

The path to lasting and powerful change to your health and weight is paved with foods that you look forward to eating and that are filling while also being low in calories. The recipes that follow are designed to be just that, and more: They're easy to prepare, make use of readily available ingredients and components you can make ahead of time, and, above all, are delicious.

Each dish has tons of flavor thanks to the creative use of spices and low-fat sauces and dressings that you can easily mix and match to keep your meals varied without having to make several recipes for each meal. You might initially feel like the servings are huge or larger than you're used to—but don't be scared! They're supposed to be; that's the beauty of eating low-calorie, high-bulk foods. If you can't finish your meal, don't force yourself. Just set it aside to have it a little later if you get hungry.

For those of you on the Precisely Plant-Based path, I've included the calorie information with each recipe so you can build your meals according to your daily calorie target if you want to. Otherwise, feel free to disregard that information, as these recipes all qualify as mindfully plant-based eating. If you're new to plant-based eating, I highly recommend following one of the meal plans in Chapter 5. This will give you a sense of all the food you'll be able to eat while still hitting your goals. As your caloric needs shift, so, too, can the recipes you reach for.

If you're on the maintenance path, you have several options because of the increased flexibility in the number of calories you're eating each day:

- Follow one of the twenty-eight-day meal plans on pages 47–50 or 53–56 and simply eat additional servings of these recipes.
- Add 1/4 avocado to your lunch or dinner; drizzle extra sauce or sprinkle condiments on your dishes; or add just a few more snacks or treats than you had previously allowed when you were eating for a calorie deficit.
- Check out What I Eat in a Week on page 63 for a snapshot of what the maintenance phase looks like in real life.

CHAPTER 7

Breakfast

Whether you eat it first thing in the morning or not until noon, breakfast sets the tone for the rest of the day. A wholesome meal that's filling and gives you steady and stable energy for the entire day (read: no major crashes, mood swings, or cravings) creates momentum for making more choices that are aligned with your goals. In other words, a healthy breakfast leads to a healthy lunch, which then leads to a healthy dinner.

Some days will be easier than others, and not every day will look exactly the way you want it to, but breakfast will always be your opportunity to hit the reset button and start fresh.

Vanilla Berry Parfait with Chocolate Granola

While some mornings I wake up craving a big, savory breakfast, other times I have a major sweet tooth. That used to mean stopping at a fast-food chain for a berry parfait, which I later learned was full of sugars, fats, and preservatives, despite its healthy-sounding name. To satisfy that sweet-tooth itch while also setting myself up for maximum satiety, I came up with this recipe. It's creamy and ice cream sundae–like with crunchy choco-latey bits from my favorite homemade granola, but it isn't loaded with the sugars, preservatives, and animal fat of a fast-food parfait.

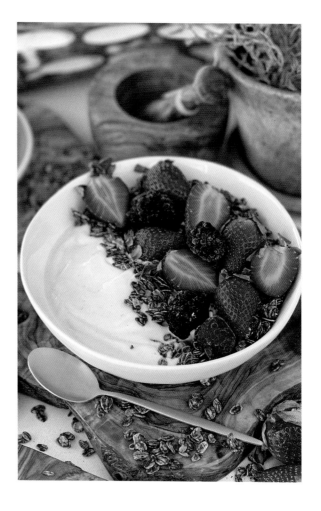

1 cup plain, unsweetened coconut yogurt (see page 34)

½ teaspoon vanilla extract

Stevia or monk fruit, to taste

2 cups fresh or frozen berries of your choice

½ cup Chocolate Granola (page 70)

In a medium bowl, stir together the yogurt and vanilla and sweeten to taste. Top with the berries and the granola.

NUTRITION FACTS
FOR 1 SERVING: **CALORIES:** 437 **PROTEIN:** 9g **CARBS:** 67g **FAT:** 11g

Chocolate Granola

MAKES

6

¼-CUP
SERVINGS

This cocoa-packed, maple-sweetened granola gives chocolate cereal vibes without all the added fat and sugar. It's delicious in a bowl with berries and a little almond milk, or as a decadent, crunchy topping for oats, fruit, yogurt, smoothies, or my Vanilla Berry Parfait (page 69).

1½ cups (122g) rolled oats
¼ cup maple syrup
2 tablespoons unsweetened cocoa powder
1 teaspoon vanilla extract

---

1. Preheat the oven to 375°F. Line a baking sheet with parchment paper and set aside.

2. In a medium bowl, combine the oats, maple syrup, cocoa powder, and vanilla. Mix well. Spread the mixture over the prepared baking sheet and bake for 10 minutes, until lightly browned.

3. Allow the granola to cool completely before storing it in an airtight container at room temperature for up to 1 week.

NUTRITION FACTS
FOR ¼ CUP: **CALORIES:** 117 **PROTEIN:** 3g **CARBS:** 21g **FAT:** 2g

Raspberry Chocolate Muffins

SERVES

2½

MAKES 10 MUFFINS

I love making a batch of muffins whenever I'm in the mood for something warm and decadent. When it comes to baked goods, making your own means you get the final say in every single ingredient, so you can indulge without any worry about what's hiding in your delicious treat. It also means you can play around with new flavor combinations, like raspberry and chocolate, which is one of my favorite ingredient marriages. But maybe best of all, you can have three muffins as one serving, which I like to enjoy with fresh fruit.

Cooking spray (see page 33)
1 cup water
1 teaspoon vanilla extract
1½ cups (180g) whole-wheat flour, or oat flour for gluten-free muffins
¼ cup (50g) sugar
1 teaspoon baking powder
¼ teaspoon sea salt
1 cup fresh raspberries
¼ cup dairy-free chocolate chips (see Note)

1. Preheat the oven to 375°F. Lightly coat 9 to 10 cups of a silicone muffin pan with cooking spray and set aside.

2. In a large mixing bowl, combine the water and vanilla. Mix in the flour, sugar, baking powder, and salt until the batter is smooth. Gently fold in the raspberries and chocolate chips until evenly distributed.

3. Divide the batter evenly among the prepared muffin cups, about ¼ cup batter per cup. Bake for 15 to 18 minutes, until a toothpick inserted into the center of a muffin comes out clean (aside from melty chocolate or raspberry).

4. Allow the muffins to cool completely before storing in an airtight container at room temperature for up to 3 days.

NOTE: If you want to save calories, omit the chocolate chips from the batter. Instead, use half the amount (2 tablespoons) to sprinkle over the top of each muffin before baking.

NUTRITION FACTS
FOR 3 MUFFINS: CALORIES: 362   PROTEIN: 9g   CARBS: 60g   FAT: 7.5g

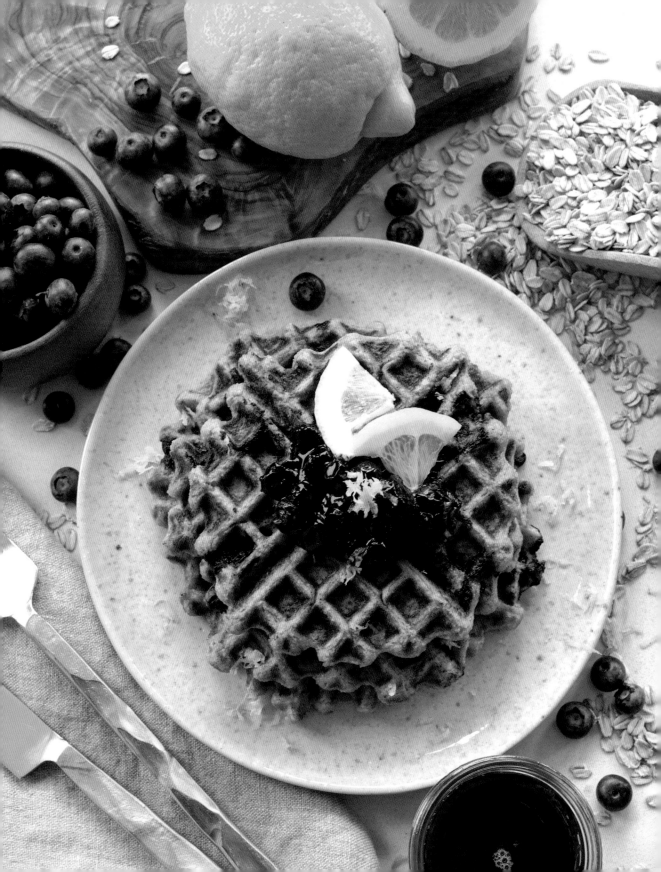

Blueberry Lemon
Oat Waffles

This recipe is inspired by all my amazing readers, who've been sharing with me that they love my gluten-free blueberry pancakes and started making them into waffles. Brilliant! For anyone who hasn't discovered this fun little hack that transforms pancakes into fluffy, chewy waffles, I wanted to create an official recipe.

Cooking spray (see page 33)

1 cup (82g) rolled oats

1 medium ripe banana (101g)

1 teaspoon vanilla extract

½ teaspoon lemon extract

½ teaspoon baking powder

Pinch of sea salt

¾ cup water

½ cup whole fresh blueberries, plus ½ cup mashed and warmed blueberries, for serving

1 tablespoon maple syrup, for serving

---

1. Preheat the waffle iron (I use a four-waffle iron for this recipe) and lightly coat it with cooking spray.

2. In a blender, combine the oats, banana, vanilla, lemon extract, baking powder, and salt. Add the water and blend until smooth. Gently fold in the ½ cup whole blueberries.

3. Pour the batter into the waffle iron, using about ¼ cup batter for each waffle. If using a four-waffle iron, you'll do this in two batches. Cook for 5 to 8 minutes or until the waffles no longer stick or pull apart. Repeat with the remaining batter and serve hot with syrup and the mashed blueberries.

NUTRITION FACTS

FOR 1 SERVING, NOT INCLUDING MAPLE SYRUP: CALORIES: 459   PROTEIN: 12g   CARBS: 77g   FAT: 6g

Strawberry Lemon Muffins

SERVES
2½
MAKES 10
MUFFINS

I love going to the farmers' market during the spring and summer to load up on ingredients to play with and to find inspiration for new dishes. One of my favorite moments of the season is when big flats of fresh-picked berries, especially strawberries, appear. I always know that I'll be able to find a good use for them—even if it's just popping them all straight into my mouth—and my most recent creation is these muffins. The lemon gives a pop of bright flavor while also accentuating the natural sweetness of the strawberries—the perfect taste of summer.

NOTE: You could also use this batter to make pancakes. Just heat a nonstick griddle and ladle in the batter as you would for flapjacks.

You can also swap in any fruit for the strawberries. Feel free to add cinnamon or other warm spices such as nutmeg or cloves, too.

Cooking spray (see page 33)

1½ cups (180g) whole-wheat flour, or oat flour for gluten-free muffins

¼ cup (50g) sugar

1 teaspoon baking powder

¼ teaspoon sea salt

1 cup water

1 teaspoon vanilla extract

1 teaspoon lemon extract

1 cup hulled and chopped fresh strawberries

1 teaspoon lemon zest

1. Preheat the oven to 375°F. Lightly coat 10 wells of a muffin tin with cooking spray and set aside.

2. In a medium bowl, whisk together the flour, sugar, baking powder, and salt. Set aside.

3. In a small bowl, stir together the water, vanilla, and lemon extract. Slowly pour the water mixture into the dry ingredients and mix until smooth. Gently fold in the strawberries and lemon zest.

4. Divide the batter among the prepared muffin cups, about ¼ cup each. Bake until a toothpick inserted into the center of a muffin comes out clean, 18 to 22 minutes.

5. Allow the muffins to cool completely before releasing from the pan. The muffins will keep in an airtight container at room temperature for up to 3 days.

NUTRITION FACTS
FOR 4 MUFFINS: CALORIES: 352 **PROTEIN:** 10g
CARBS: 68g **FAT:** 2.5g

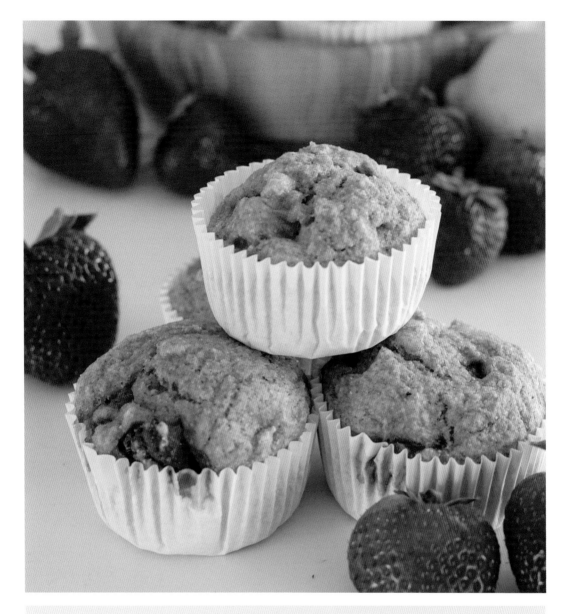

Variations

Try these other delicious flavor combinations:

- ½ tablespoon poppy seeds + 1 teaspoon lemon extract + 1 teaspoon lemon zest

- 1 cup fresh or frozen blueberries + 1 teaspoon lemon extract + 1 teaspoon lemon zest

- 1 cup fresh or frozen raspberries + 1 teaspoon orange extract + 1 teaspoon orange zest

- 1 cup fresh or frozen sliced peaches + 1 teaspoon orange extract + 1 teaspoon orange zest

Raspberry Lemon Poppy Seed Pancakes

SERVES

2

MAKES 10 PANCAKES

If I had to choose my all-time favorite breakfast foods, it would be a dead heat between lemon poppy seed muffins and pancakes. So, when I was thinking about fun ways to work new offerings into my breakfast rotation, I thought, Why not create a mash-up between the two and make them healthy? For even more flavor—and a good dose of fiber and phytonutrients—I've also added raspberries into the mix.

1¼ cups (150g) whole-wheat flour, or oat flour for gluten-free pancakes

2 tablespoons (25g) sugar

2 teaspoons baking powder

½ teaspoon sea salt

1¼ cups water

1 teaspoon vanilla extract

1 teaspoon lemon extract

1 teaspoon lemon zest

½ tablespoon poppy seeds

1 cup fresh raspberries, halved, plus more for serving (optional)

Cooking spray (see page 33, optional)

Maple syrup, for serving

---

1. In a medium bowl, whisk together the flour, sugar, baking powder, and salt. Set aside.

2. In a small bowl, stir together the water, vanilla, and lemon extract. While stirring, slowly pour the water mixture into the dry ingredients and mix until smooth. Gently fold in the lemon zest, poppy seeds, and raspberries.

3. Heat a large nonstick skillet over medium-high heat. If you like, you can coat it with cooking spray to encourage even cooking, but it's not necessary. Working in batches, use a ¼-cup scoop to portion the batter into the pan. Cook until the bottom of the pancake is light gold, 2 to 3 minutes. Flip and repeat on the other side. Repeat with the remaining batter and serve the pancakes hot topped with raspberries and syrup, if desired.

NUTRITION FACTS

FOR 1 SERVING (5 PANCAKES), NOT INCLUDING MAPLE SYRUP: **CALORIES:** 360   **PROTEIN:** 11g   **CARBS:** 63g   **FAT:** 3g

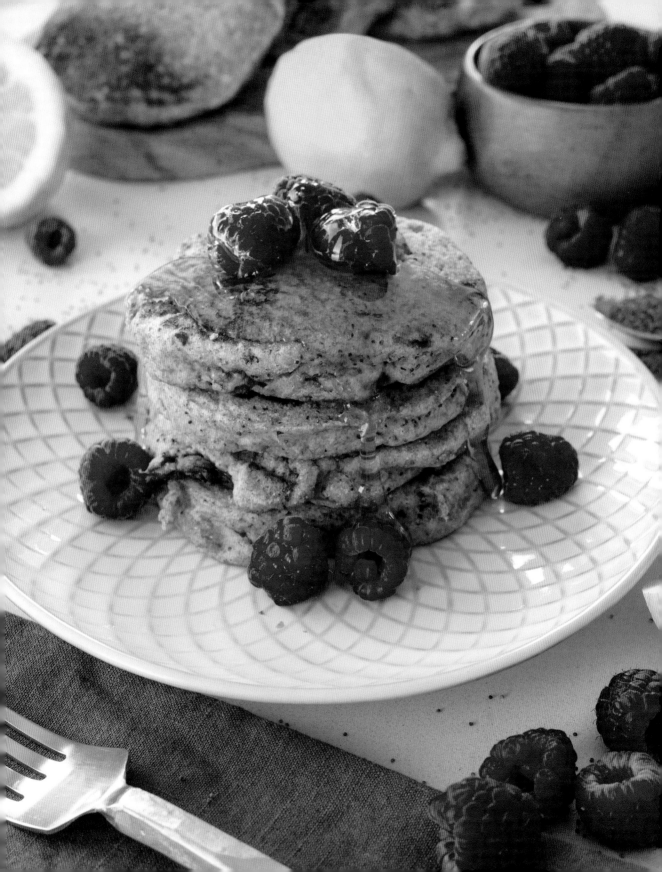

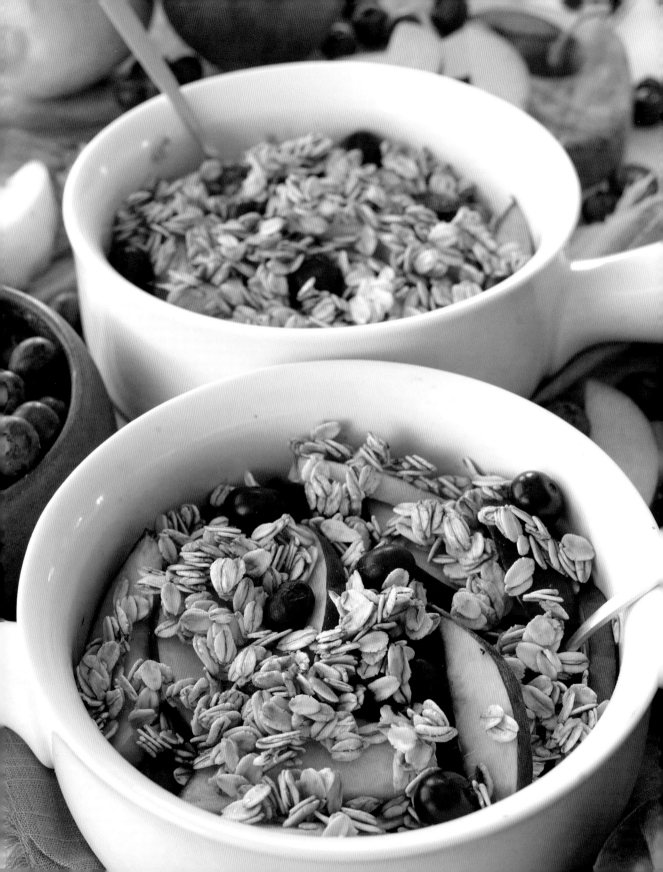

Blueberry Peach Crisp

SERVES
2

Every summer we're lucky enough to have an abundance of fresh blueberries and peaches from our orchard. Just like most fruits and veggies that come into season together, these two taste amazing when combined—especially when baked into a simple and satisfying crisp. Oh, and did I mention that we're talking breakfast and not dessert here? Just wait until you see how a maple-infused oat topping makes syrupy baked fruit taste like it could easily be an after-dinner treat (which it could also be!). Don't be tempted to skip the almond extract; it adds a unique and subtle cherry-like flavor that gives this dish even more depth.

1. Preheat the oven to 375°F.

2. Make the filling: In a medium bowl, toss together the blueberries, peaches, lemon juice, and vanilla. Divide the mixture between two 6 x 8-inch dishes. Set aside.

3. Make the topping: In a medium bowl, mix together the oats, maple syrup, vanilla, and almond extract. Divide the mixture evenly and top the two dishes of fruit. Bake for 20 minutes, until the fruit is bubbling and the topping is golden brown.

FOR THE FILLING
4 cups (300g) fresh or frozen
and thawed blueberries

4 peaches (350g), sliced, or 4 cups
thawed frozen peach slices

4 tablespoons fresh lemon juice

4 teaspoons vanilla extract

FOR THE TOPPING
1 cup (41g) rolled oats

2 tablespoons maple syrup

1 teaspoon vanilla extract

½ teaspoon almond extract

NUTRITION FACTS
FOR 1 SERVING: CALORIES: 543   PROTEIN: 11g   CARBS: 102g   FAT: 2g

Breakfast Salad

SERVES
1

When I started looking for ways to incorporate more greens into my life other than in smoothies and savory salads, a mind-blowing idea came to me: "the Breakfast Salad." I saw it as a perfect way to combine lots of fresh fruit and all those nutritious greens—almost like a deconstructed smoothie. Here I use either white beans or chickpeas, which have a mild flavor that pairs well with both sweet and savory ingredients and give the dish a hearty boost. The citrus poppy seed dressing pulls everything together, and if you've prepped it ahead of time, this dish comes together very quickly.

1. Make the dressing: In a small bowl, mix together the orange juice, lime juice, maple syrup or sweetener of your choice, and poppy seeds. Set aside.

2. Make the salad: In a large bowl, create a bed of the greens and top with the peach slices, strawberries, and blueberries. Top with the beans or chickpeas, if using, and sprinkle with the mint, if using. Drizzle with the dressing (I use all of it) and toss to coat.

FOR THE CITRUS POPPY SEED DRESSING
¼ cup fresh orange juice

1 tablespoon fresh lime juice

1 teaspoon maple syrup or other sweetener of your choice

¼ teaspoon poppy seeds

FOR THE SALAD
4 cups spring greens or other greens you like

1 peach, pit removed and sliced

1 cup hulled and chopped strawberries

¾ cup blueberries

1 cup (260g) cooked or canned white beans or chickpeas (drained and rinsed if canned); optional

1 tablespoon chopped fresh mint leaves (optional)

NUTRITION FACTS
FOR 1 SERVING, INCLUDING WHITE BEANS: CALORIES: 456   PROTEIN: 21g   CARBS: 68g   FAT: 1.7g

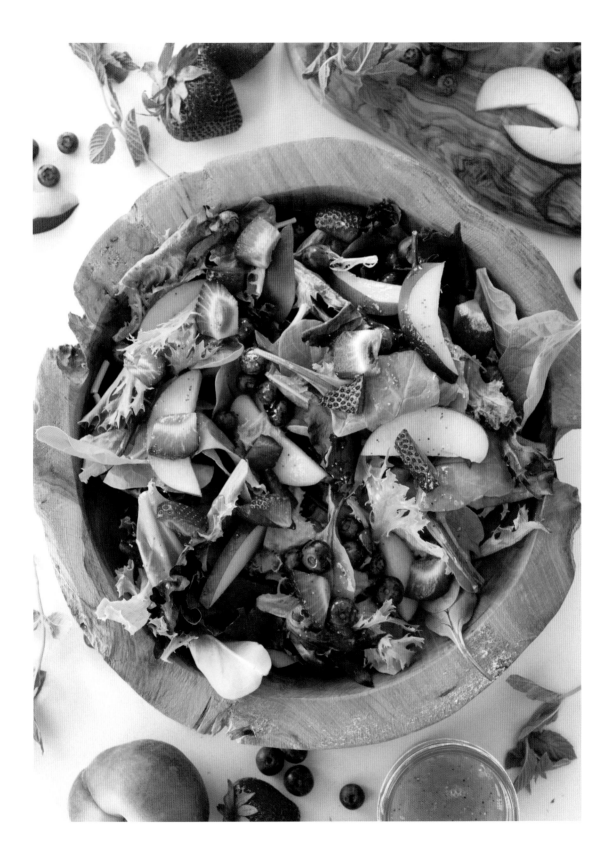

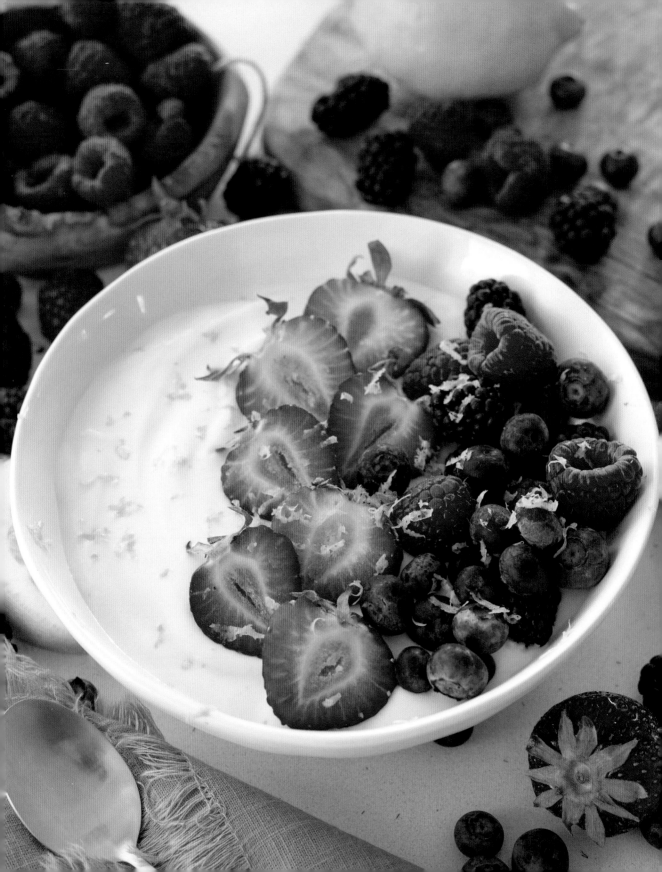

Lemon Berry Patch Yogurt

SERVES
1

When I first started playing around with creating a calorie deficit, one of the first places I looked to eliminate calories was in sweeteners. But finding flavored yogurt devoid of sugar was a challenge. While there are a ton of plant-based yogurt options at the store, which is great, many of them are full of added sugar. Luckily, it couldn't be easier to enhance your own yogurt by starting with a base of unsweetened plant-based yogurt, sweetening it with stevia or monk fruit, and then loading it up with all your favorite mix-ins.

In a medium bowl, stir together the yogurt and lemon extract. Adjust the flavor with more lemon extract, if desired, and sweeten to taste. Top with the berries and enjoy.

1½ cups plain, unsweetened coconut yogurt (see page 34)

½ teaspoon lemon extract, plus more to taste

Stevia or monk fruit sweetener, to taste

1½ cups sliced strawberries

¾ cup fresh or frozen and defrosted raspberries

¾ cup fresh or frozen and defrosted blueberries

¾ cup fresh or frozen and defrosted blackberries

NUTRITION FACTS
FOR 1 SERVING: CALORIES: 389 PROTEIN: 6g CARBS: 48g FAT: 13g

Chocolate Peanut Butter Oatmeal

SERVES
1

Not only will this recipe scratch the itch for a sweet, indulgent breakfast every time with its combination of creamy oats, chocolate chips, and peanut butter but I've also snuck in some cauliflower for good measure. That's right—that versatile, mild-tasting veggie is perfect for folding into this decadent creation because it adds belly-filling, sustaining bulk and fiber. You'd never guess it's there, and yet you're reaping all the benefits of this nutritional powerhouse, such as its ample choline, which is essential for healthy nervous system function and memory.

1½ cups plus 1 tablespoon water
¾ cup rolled oats
½ cup frozen riced cauliflower
¼ teaspoon vanilla extract, plus more to taste
Stevia or monk fruit, to taste
2 tablespoons powdered peanut butter
2 tablespoons dairy-free chocolate chips

1. In a medium pot, combine 1½ cups of the water with the oats and riced cauliflower. Bring the mixture to a boil over medium-high heat, stirring occasionally, and immediately reduce to a simmer. Continue cooking and stirring until the oats are tender, 3 to 5 minutes.

2. Stir in the vanilla and sweeten to taste with the stevia or monk fruit and more vanilla, if desired.

3. In a small bowl, stir together the powdered peanut butter and the remaining 1 tablespoon of water until smooth.

4. Top the oats with the peanut butter and the chocolate chips and enjoy.

NOTE: If you want to reduce the number of calories in this recipe, you can use one tablespoon of chocolate chips instead of two. You'd be amazed at how much chocolatey flavor you can get from just that amount once it gets all melted and gooey.

NUTRITION FACTS
FOR 1 SERVING: CALORIES: 455   PROTEIN: 17g   CARBS: 56g   FAT: 15g

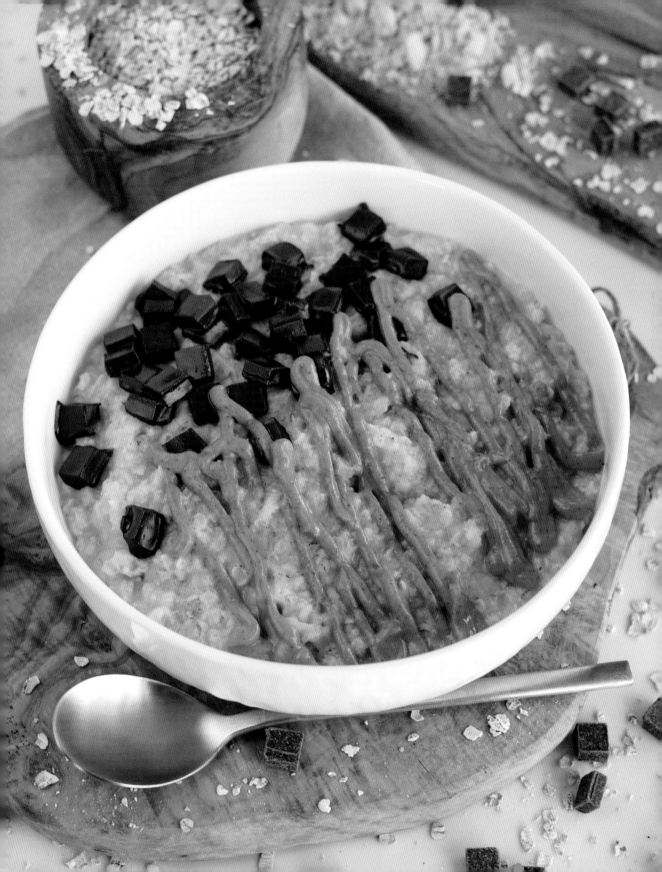

Pineapple Ginger Smoothie

MAKES
1
SMOOTHIE

I always feel good about myself when I have this smoothie. I know that the combination of spinach, ginger, and fruit won't spike my blood sugar, which many smoothies can do; plus, these ingredients are inflammation fighters. What's more, the fiber-rich ingredients will satisfy me until my next meal. I mean, if you're already getting in your greens before you've even started your day, I consider that a big win.

---

2 medium bananas (236g)
1½ cups (280g) frozen pineapple
2 handfuls of spinach
½-inch piece of ginger, peeled
1 cup plain, unsweetened almond milk

In a blender, combine the bananas, pineapple, spinach, ginger, and almond milk. Blend until smooth.

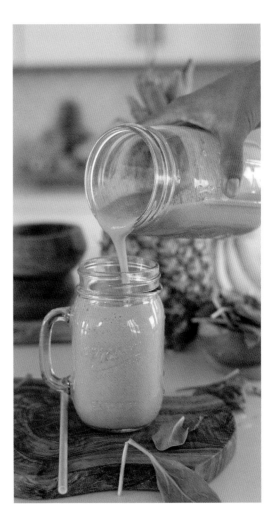

NUTRITION FACTS
FOR 1 SMOOTHIE: CALORIES: 436   PROTEIN: 8g   CARBS: 86g   FAT: 3.5g

Chocolate Peanut Butter Smoothie

MAKES
1
SMOOTHIE

Sometimes you just feel like dessert for breakfast, and this chocolatey, peanut buttery smoothie hits the spot without sabotaging your day or your progress. Who doesn't love the peace of mind of knowing that something so decadent is also nourishing your body with wholesome ingredients?

---

2 medium bananas (236g)
1 cup plain, unsweetened almond milk
½ cup (41g) rolled oats
2 tablespoons (12g) powdered peanut butter
1 tablespoon unsweetened cocoa powder
½ teaspoon vanilla extract

In a blender, combine the bananas, almond milk, oats, powdered peanut butter, cocoa powder, vanilla, and ½ to 1 cup ice cubes. Blend until smooth.

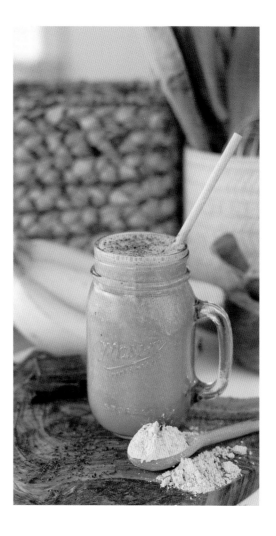

NUTRITION FACTS
FOR 1 SMOOTHIE: CALORIES: 468 **PROTEIN:** 15g **CARBS:** 78g **FAT:** 8g

Coffee Caramel Smoothie

Iced coffee lover? Say no more! I've got you covered with a smoothie that hits like your favorite sweet morning drink but without the cream and sugar. Instead, frozen bananas and Medjool dates deliver decadent creaminess with a rich, caramel flavor. You won't miss the drive-through or the blood sugar spike and ensuing crash from the highly processed fast-food version.

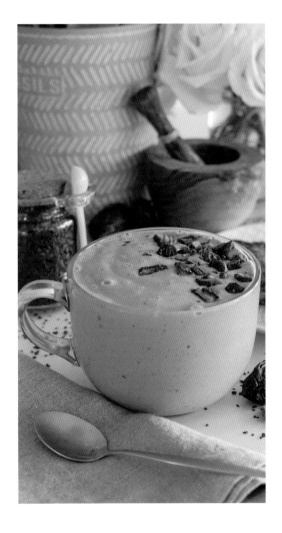

3 medium frozen bananas (354g), roughly chopped

1½ cups plain, unsweetened almond milk

2 Medjool dates, pitted, plus ½ Medjool date, pitted and chopped, for serving (optional) (48g)

2 teaspoons instant coffee (decaf, if preferred), plus more to taste (if you want stronger coffee flavor)

½ teaspoon vanilla extract

1 teaspoon dairy-free chocolate chips, for serving (optional)

In a high-speed blender, combine the bananas, almond milk, Medjool dates, instant coffee, and vanilla. Blend until smooth. Top with the chopped date and chocolate chips, if desired.

NUTRITION FACTS

FOR 1 SMOOTHIE (EXCLUDING OPTIONAL DATE AND CHOCOLATE TOPPING):   CALORIES: 502   PROTEIN: 6g
CARBS: 108g   FAT: 5g

Citrus Dragon Fruit Smoothie Bowl

MAKES
1
SMOOTHIE
BOWL

If you want more disease-fighting, immune-boosting antioxidants in your diet—and, really, who doesn't?—then this is the breakfast for you. Dragon fruit and blueberries are two highly antioxidant-rich foods, and I've combined them both in this vibrant bowl. I love reaching for a smoothie bowl when I'm looking for something as quick and easy as a smoothie to throw together but want to take a little more time to sit and savor my meal. It's especially satisfying to know that food can be as beautiful as it is nourishing.

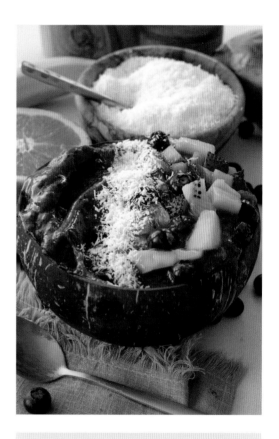

---

2 medium frozen bananas (236g),
chopped (see Note)

1 cup frozen dragon fruit, chopped

½ cup frozen blueberries

1 cup fresh orange juice

½ cup your favorite berries

1 teaspoon unsweetened shredded coconut

---

1. In a high-speed blender, combine the bananas, dragon fruit, frozen blueberries, and orange juice and blend until smooth. The mixture will be thick—more like ice cream than a smoothie you sip.

2. Transfer the smoothie to a bowl and top with the berries and shredded coconut.

NOTE: If you don't have a high-speed blender like a Blendtec or a Vitamix, you can use a food processor instead. If you only have a regular countertop blender, you may want to use bananas that haven't been frozen. Don't worry—it will still be delicious and creamy!

NUTRITION FACTS
FOR 1 SERVING: **CALORIES:** 426 **PROTEIN:** 6g **CARBS:** 90g **FAT:** 3g

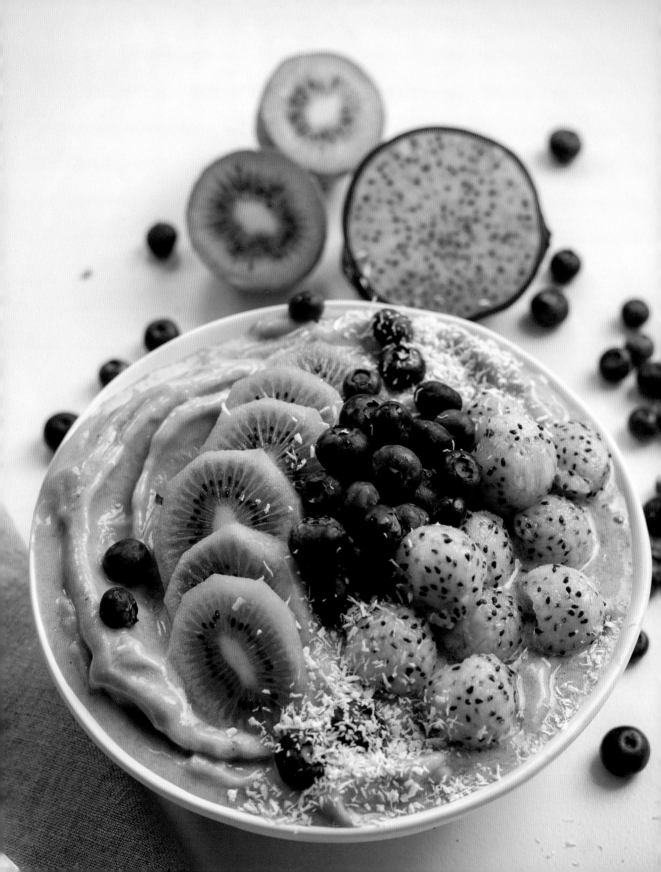

Mermaid Smoothie Bowl

MAKES

1

SMOOTHIE
BOWL

Between its tropical fruit, coconut, and ocean-blue color, this bowl gives me a major vacation moment. It's almost like having a virgin piña colada for breakfast. But it's not just another pretty dish—that beautiful hue is thanks to spirulina, a type of algae that packs tons of vitamins E, C, and B_6, in addition to phycocyanin and beta carotene, which, when combined, have powerful anti-inflammatory properties.

1. In a high-speed blender, combine the bananas, pineapple, spirulina, coconut extract (if using), and almond milk and blend until smooth. The mixture will be thick—you'll need a spoon because it's more like ice cream than a smoothie you sip.

2. Transfer the smoothie to a bowl and top with the kiwi, dragon fruit, blueberries, and coconut.

FOR THE SMOOTHIE

2 medium frozen bananas (236g), chopped (see Note)

1½ cups frozen pineapple

½ teaspoon blue spirulina powder

¼ teaspoon coconut extract (optional)

1 cup plain, unsweetened almond milk

FOR THE TOPPINGS

1 kiwi, sliced

½ cup sliced dragon fruit

½ cup blueberries

1 tablespoon unsweetened shredded coconut

NOTE: If you don't have a high-speed blender like a Blendtec or a Vitamix, you can use a food processor. If you only have a regular countertop blender, you may want to use bananas that haven't been frozen. Don't worry—it will still be delicious and creamy!

NUTRITION FACTS

FOR 1 SERVING: CALORIES: 559   PROTEIN: 9g   CARBS: 109g   FAT: 7g

Fruit Salsa with Cinnamon Toast

SERVES

1

As a '90s teen, I was addicted to a certain crunchy, sugary, cinnamon-flavored cereal. I was actually obsessed with it well into adulthood! When I started making healthier food choices, it pained me that I had to give up one of my favorite treats. Instead, I figured out a way to enjoy the same flavors and satisfying crunch of Cinnamon Toast Crunch in a more health-promoting way in this cinnamon toast and fruit salsa. The toast scratches that sweet, crunchy itch, while the fruit medley delivers all the belly-filling nutrition you want in your first meal of the day.

1. Make the fruit salsa: In a medium bowl, combine the fruit and gently toss to mix well. Set aside.

2. Make the cinnamon toast: Use a toaster or toaster oven to toast the bread to your preferred doneness. Meanwhile, in a small bowl, mix together the sugar and cinnamon. When the bread is done, sprinkle both slices with the cinnamon-sugar mixture.

3. Slice the toast into squares and top each with a mound of the fruit salsa.

NOTE: For a fun breakfast salad, heap this salsa on top of fresh greens. You can also feel free to mix and match any fruit you like here to total 3 cups.

FOR THE FRUIT SALSA
1 cup chopped strawberries
1 cup diced mango
½ cup blueberries
½ cup diced kiwi

FOR THE CINNAMON TOAST
2 slices of sprouted whole-grain bread (see page 33)
1 teaspoon sugar
¼ teaspoon ground cinnamon

NUTRITION FACTS

FOR 1 SERVING: CALORIES: 438   PROTEIN: 12g   CARBS: 82g   FAT: 3g

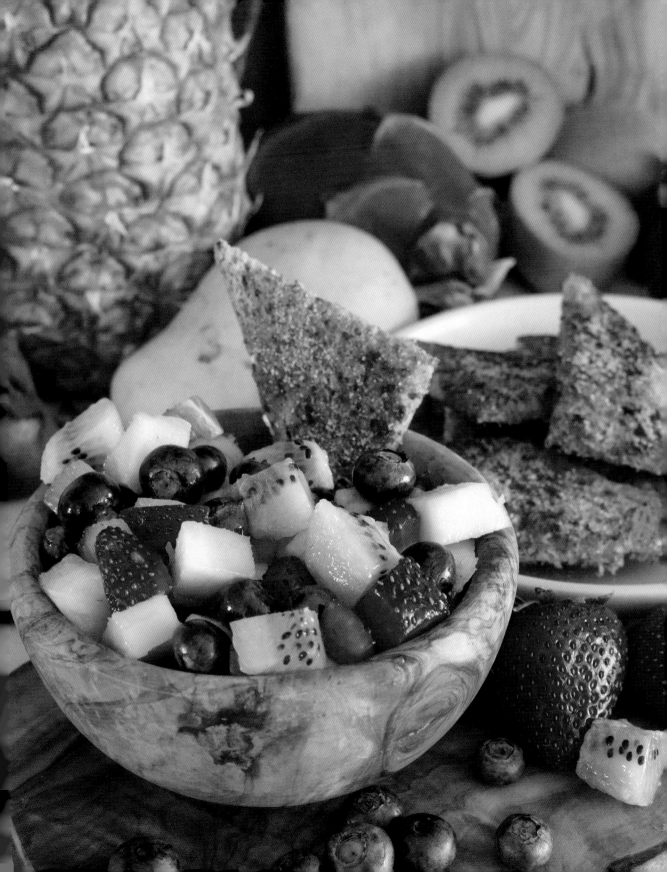

PB & J
Smoothie

MAKES
1
SMOOTHIE

My favorite smoothie place in downtown Fort Collins, Colorado, is an adorable spot called Nékter Juice Bar, where they serve the best flavor combinations. My go-to order is a peanut butter and jelly bowl, which brings me back to the classic sandwiches on white bread that I had growing up. Since I can't always make it to the shop to have my favorite bowl, I figured out how to re-create it at home so I can enjoy it anytime. Now it's at the top of my list as a favorite breakfast or snack.

4 tablespoons powdered peanut butter (see page 34)
½ cup plus 2½ tablespoons water
2 medium bananas (236g)
1½ cups frozen strawberries
1 cup frozen raspberries
½ teaspoon chia seeds (optional)
1 teaspoon unsweetened shredded coconut (optional)

1. In a small bowl, combine the powdered peanut butter with 2½ tablespoons of the water. Stir together until smooth. Set aside.

2. In a blender, combine the bananas, strawberries, raspberries, and remaining ½ cup of water. Blend until smooth.

3. Pour the mixture into a large glass jar. Top with the peanut butter, chia seeds (if using), and shredded coconut (if using) and enjoy.

NOTE: I like dolloping the peanut butter on top of this smoothie and using my spoon to grab little bits of everything with each bite, but you could also just blend the reconstituted peanut butter into the smoothie base.

NUTRITION FACTS
FOR 1 SERVING, INCLUDING CHIA SEEDS AND SHREDDED COCONUT: CALORIES: 533   PROTEIN: 22g
CARBS: 79g   FAT: 8g

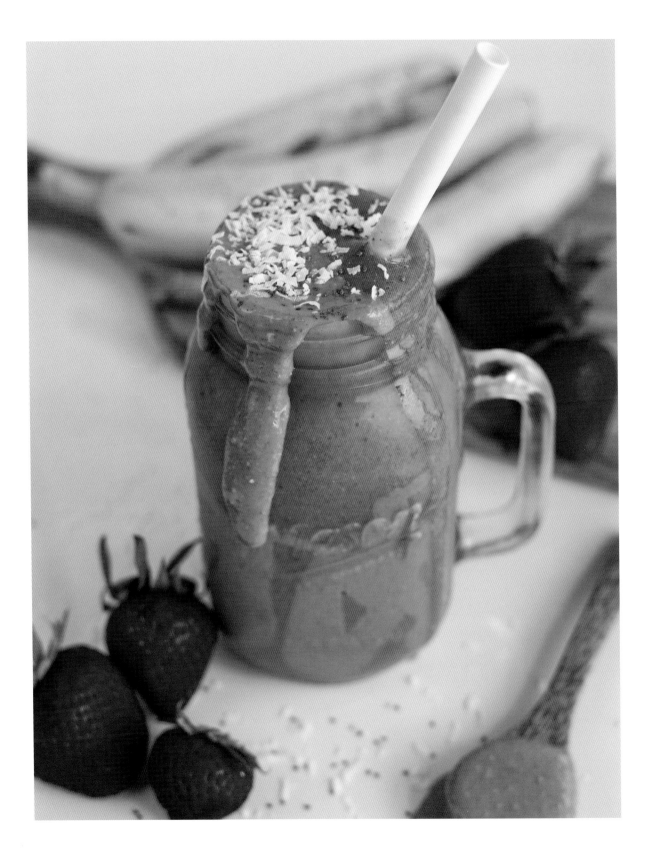

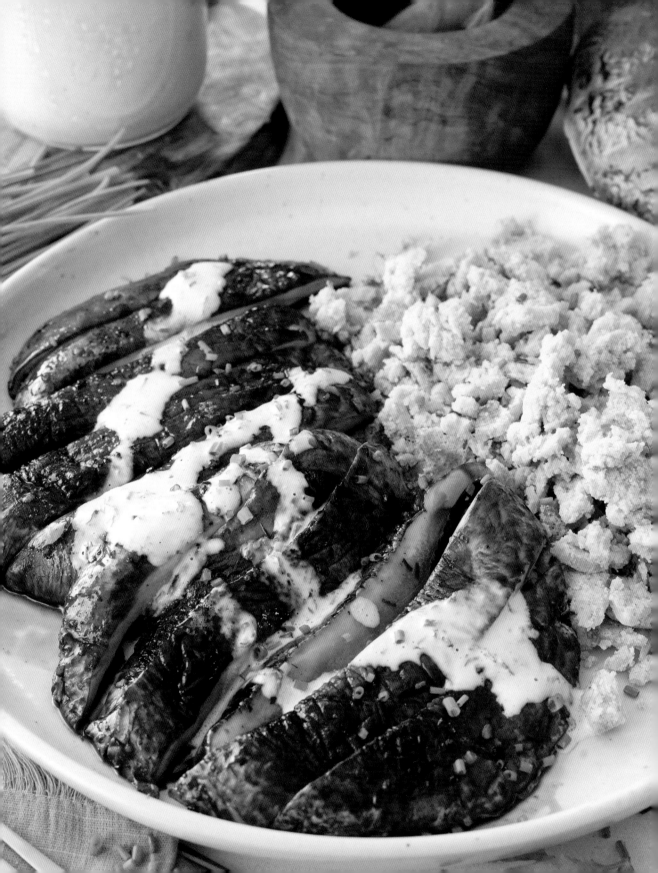

Mushroom Steak and "Eggs" with Herby Caesar

SERVES
1

I'm a big-time mushroom lover. Between their earthy, savory flavor, meaty texture, and high-fiber, low-calorie nutritional profile, it's hard to find a reason not to work them into at least one meal of the day. That's why I immediately thought of mushrooms when trying to come up with a plant-based play on classic steak and eggs. This dish is hearty and filling, and, of course, has a fraction of the dietary fat of the original.

FOR THE STEAKS
¼ cup vegan Worcestershire sauce

¼ cup water

1 teaspoon minced garlic

¼ teaspoon liquid smoke

⅛ teaspoon onion powder

Freshly ground black pepper, to taste

2 large portobello mushroom caps
(8 ounces), wiped clean

Cooking spray (see page 33, optional)

FOR SERVING
3 Garden Vegetable Chickpea Omelets
(page 98), warmed (see Note)

5 tablespoons Lemon-Herb Caesar (page 198)

Minced fresh chives, for garnish

---

1. Make the steaks: In a shallow bowl, whisk together the Worcestershire sauce, water, garlic, liquid smoke, onion powder, and a couple of twists of black pepper. Add the mushrooms and toss to coat with the marinade. Let the mushrooms marinate at room temperature for 10 minutes.

2. Heat a large nonstick skillet over medium-high heat. If you like, coat it with cooking spray to encourage the mushrooms to brown, but it isn't necessary. Add the mushrooms, top side down, and cook until they begin to brown, 3 to 5 minutes. If they start to stick, you can add a splash of water. Flip and repeat on the other side. Set aside.

3. Assemble: Chop the omelets so they resemble scrambled eggs. Slice the mushrooms and arrange them over the eggs, then drizzle with the dressing and garnish with chives.

> NOTE: This is a great way to use up leftover Garden Vegetable Chickpea Omelets, or you could prepare extra omelets to keep in the fridge just for this dish.

NUTRITION FACTS
FOR 1 SERVING: CALORIES: 367   PROTEIN: 16g   CARBS: 41g   FAT: 12g

Garden Vegetable Chickpea Omelet

SERVES
1
MAKES 3
OMELETS

Going out for breakfast on the weekends used to be one of my favorite things, but trying to find restaurants that offer plant-based options other than oatmeal was frustrating. So, I decided to take matters into my own hands, and I created a restaurant-style omelet to enjoy in the comfort of my own home. It's full of fiber-packed vegetables (seriously, add as many as you want, and in any combination); it packs a ton of protein thanks to the chickpea base; and it doesn't have anywhere near the amount of fat and grease that omelets from a restaurant kitchen contain. Topped with avocado and plenty of hot sauce or salsa, this is easily one of my favorite savory morning meals.

---

1 cup (92g) chickpea flour
1 cup water
¼ teaspoon garlic powder
⅛ teaspoon onion powder
½ teaspoon black salt or sea salt (see Note)
Pinch of turmeric (optional, for color)
Cooking spray (see page 33, optional)
Assorted veggies (see Note)
Garlic salt, to taste
¼ medium avocado (25g)
Your favorite salsa and/or hot sauce, for serving

NUTRITION FACTS
FOR 1 SERVING (3 OMELETS), NOT INCLUDING AVOCADO
(AVOCADO ADDS 40 CALORIES): CALORIES: 359
PROTEIN: 21g CARBS: 44g FAT: 6g

1. In a medium bowl, whisk together the chickpea flour, water, garlic powder, onion powder, black or sea salt, and turmeric (if using). The omelet batter should be smooth. Set aside.

2. Heat a large nonstick skillet over medium-high heat. If you like, you can coat it with cooking spray to encourage even cooking, but it isn't necessary. Add the veggies with a pinch of garlic salt and cook until tender. The timing will depend on the vegetables you choose and how many there are. If the veggies start to stick, you can add a splash of water to the pan to loosen them. Transfer the veggies to a plate or bowl and wipe out the pan.

3. If desired, coat the pan again with cooking spray and place over medium heat. Scoop the batter into the pan using a ½-cup measuring cup. Use the bottom of the measuring cup to gently spread the batter until it resembles a large pancake about 6 inches in diameter and ¼ inch thick. Cook the omelet until the bottom starts to brown and it's no longer wet in the center, about 3 minutes. Flip and continue cooking until the other side is lightly golden and set, about another 3 minutes. Transfer the omelet to a plate and repeat with the remaining batter.

4. Divide the veggies among the omelets and top with avocado, salsa, and/or hot sauce. Serve immediately.

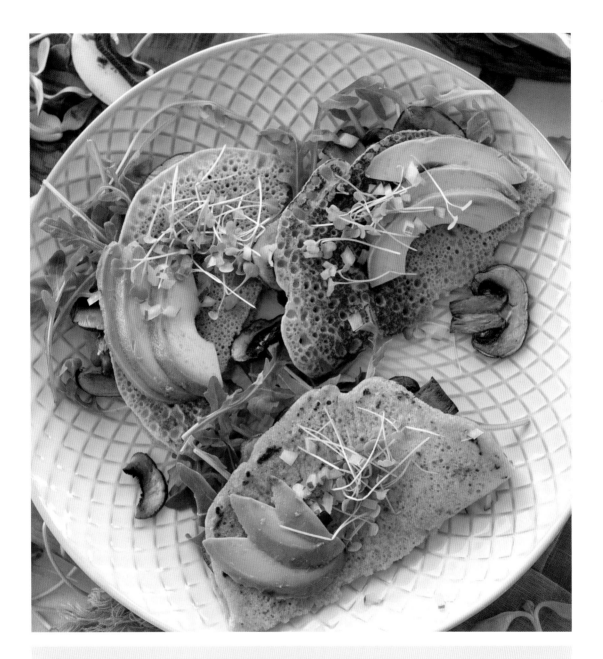

NOTE: This mixture is better suited for smaller omelets, which is why a serving contains three of them. You can also use any leftovers with other recipes (such as Mushroom Steak and "Eggs" with Herby Caesar on page 97 or Gardener's Breakfast on page 105). For the filling, the sky really is the limit; feel free to use as many veggies as you like and play around with combinations that suit your taste and mood. Aim for at least 2 cups. My favorite options are sliced mushrooms, diced onions, diced bell peppers, diced tomatoes, chopped greens, and sprouts. I call for using black salt here because it has a naturally eggy flavor that makes it feel like you're really eating a plate of eggs, but sea salt will work just fine.

Asian-Inspired Vegetable Pancakes

SERVES
2

I love my smoothies, but most mornings I'm in the mood for something savory—and no one said that you couldn't make a dish for breakfast that could also work for lunch or dinner. I consistently find myself reaching for this recipe, which is a play on a Chinese scallion pancake studded with loads of vegetables and topped off with a bright, salty soy sauce–based dressing.

FOR THE BATTER

1½ cups (237g) white rice flour
¾ cup (90g) tapioca flour
½ teaspoon sea salt
½ teaspoon garlic powder
½ teaspoon onion powder
Pinch of turmeric (optional, for color)
1¾ cups water

FOR ASSEMBLY

5 ounces shiitake mushrooms, wiped clean, stems removed, and thinly sliced
1 cup thinly sliced red bell pepper
1 cup thinly sliced zucchini
½ cup sliced scallions (white and green parts)
Cooking spray (see page 33, optional)
3 tablespoons All-Purpose Asian Dressing (page 194), optional

1. Make the batter: In a medium bowl, whisk together the white rice flour, tapioca flour, salt, garlic powder, onion powder, and turmeric (if using). Add the water and whisk until the batter is smooth. It will be on the thinner side, similar to crepe batter. Set aside.

2. Assemble the pancakes: In a medium bowl, toss together the mushrooms, pepper, zucchini, and scallions.

3. Heat a 10-inch nonstick skillet over medium-high heat. If you like, you can coat it with cooking spray to help the pancakes cook evenly, but it isn't necessary. Add about ½ cup of the veggies to the pan and spread them out evenly. Give the batter a stir (the rice flour likes to settle at the bottom of the bowl), then pour ½ cup of the batter over the vegetables, making sure they're covered. Let the pancake cook for 5 minutes, or until the edges begin to brown and the pancake is no longer runny on top. Use a large spatula to gently flip the pancake and cook for another 3 to 5 minutes, until lightly golden and set.

4. Transfer the pancake to a plate and repeat with the remaining vegetables and pancake batter (you'll most likely run out of vegetables first). You should end up with 5½ pancakes; you can save the extra 1½ pancakes for a snack. Enjoy them warmed up or at room temperature, drizzled with dressing, if desired.

NUTRITION FACTS
FOR 1 SERVING (2 PANCAKES), NOT INCLUDING DRESSING:
CALORIES: 472 PROTEIN: 8g CARBS: 101g FAT: 2g

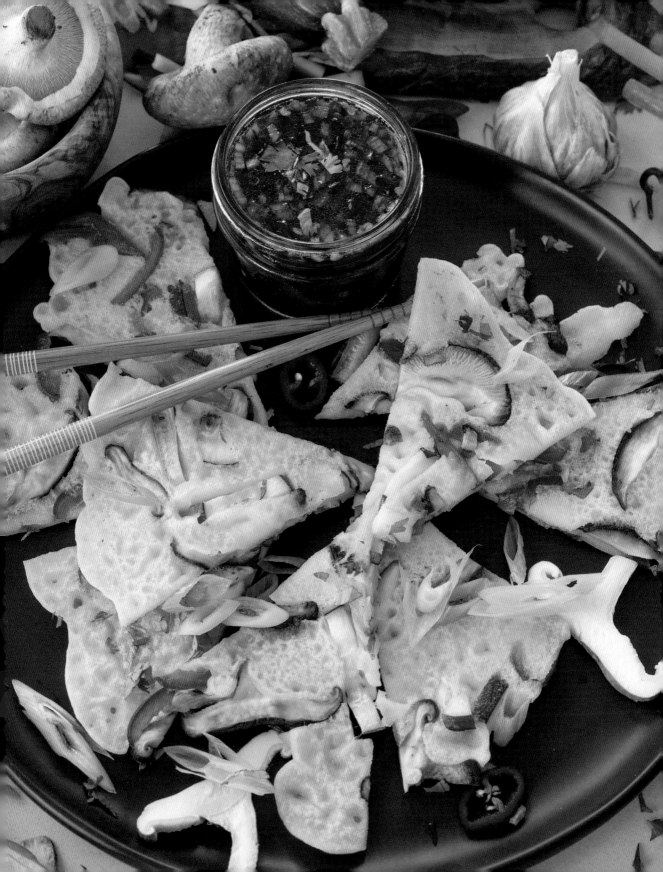

Garlic Herb Potato Waffles

SERVES
1
MAKES 3
WAFFLES

The humble potato is pretty much what enabled me to heal my relationship with food. Eating carbohydrates in their many whole, plant-based forms finally helped me see that there's no such thing as a "bad" plant—potatoes included! They're filling and full of carbohydrate energy, not to mention the fact that they're crazy delicious when treated right. This recipe is where creamy, garlicky mashed potatoes meet the crispness of French fries, and what a heavenly combination it is. It's also a great way to use up leftover cooked potatoes, and it's a handy make-ahead meal.

2 medium to large Yukon Gold potatoes (550g)

2 teaspoons dried rosemary

1 teaspoon garlic powder

½ teaspoon onion powder

½ teaspoon dried thyme

½ teaspoon sea salt

Cooking spray (see page 33)

3 tablespoons Lemon-Herb Caesar (page 198), Smokehouse Ranch (page 197), or Pimento Cheese Sauce (page 225), optional

1. Boil or bake your potatoes with the skin on. If baking, preheat the oven to 425°F. Pierce the potatoes all over and bake on a baking sheet for 45 minutes, until fork tender. If boiling, cut the potatoes into 1-inch cubes and put in a medium or large pot. Add just enough water to cover the potatoes, put on the lid, and bring to a boil over medium-high heat. Boil for 20 to 25 minutes, until fork tender. If using an Instant Pot, insert the steaming basket and add the potatoes. Add just enough water to cover and put on the lid. Use the Steam function to cook for 18 minutes. Release the pressure manually.

2. Allow the potatoes to cool and preheat a waffle iron to high heat.

3. When the potatoes are cool enough to handle, place them in a medium bowl with the rosemary, garlic powder, onion powder, thyme, and salt. Use a potato masher or fork to mash the potatoes until just about smooth (some lumps are okay) and evenly combine the seasonings.

4. Lightly coat the waffle iron with cooking spray. Form one-third of the potato mixture into a patty and place it in the waffle iron. Cook for 5 to 10 minutes, or until crispy. Transfer the finished waffle to a plate and repeat with the remaining potato mixture. You should end up with 3 waffles.

5. Enjoy warm and drizzled with the sauce of your choice.

NUTRITION FACTS
FOR 1 SERVING (3 WAFFLES) WITHOUT DRESSING:
CALORIES: 433   **PROTEIN:** 10g   **CARBS:** 88g   **FAT:** 1g

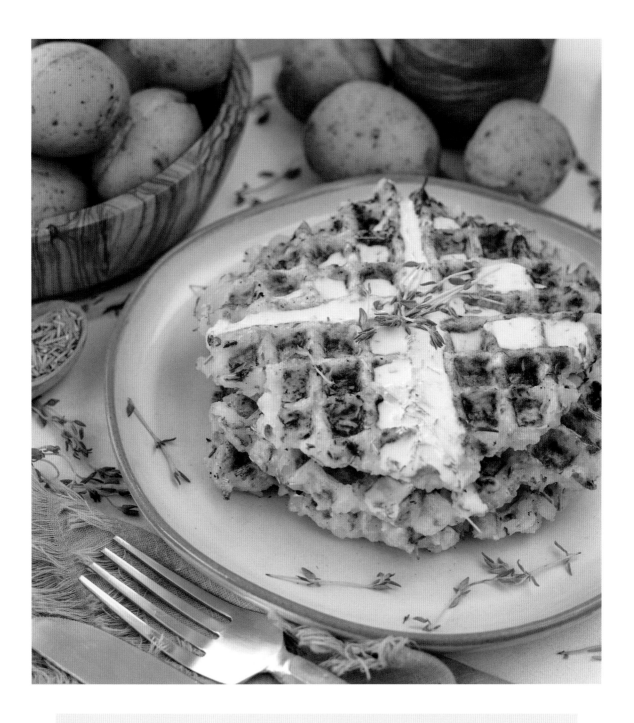

NOTE: I like to scale up this recipe so I can keep a batch of these in the fridge. When I'm ready to enjoy them, I pop them in the oven or the air fryer (about 425°F for 5 minutes for each method) to crisp them back up.

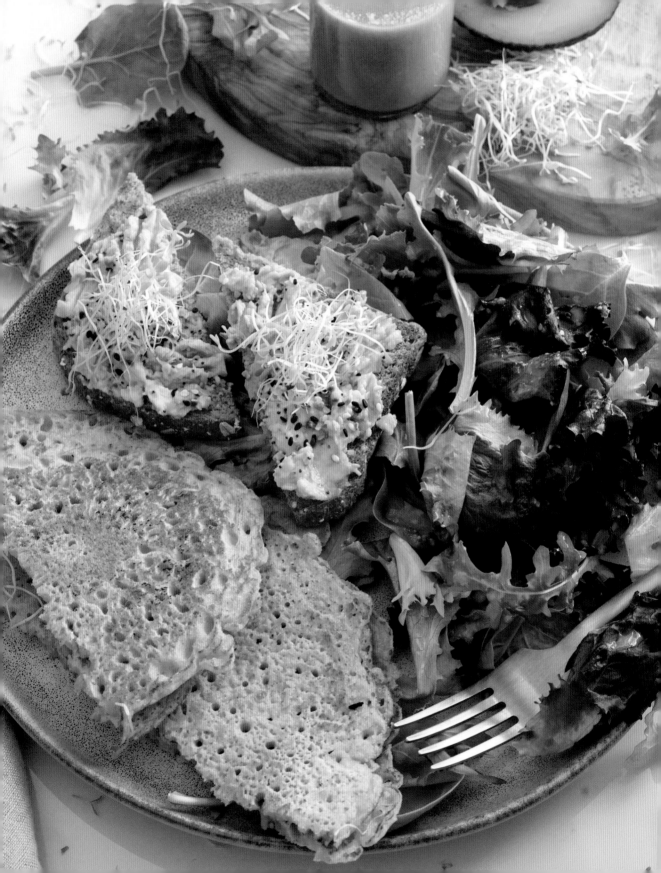

Gardener's Breakfast

SERVES
1

Whenever we're in Denver, my husband and I like to have breakfast at a little vegetarian café called the Corner Beet. I always order the same thing: the Farmer's Table. It's essentially greens tossed with a simple vinaigrette, plus "eggs" (or chickpea omelets, in this case) and avocado toast, which isn't exactly a revolutionary idea, but it is simple, creamy, and so, so tasty. It manages to feel satisfying and nourishing yet light—like you're heading out to spend some time in the garden.

½ tablespoon maple syrup

½ tablespoon fresh lemon juice

½ tablespoon Dijon mustard

3 cups spring greens

2 Garden Vegetable Chickpea Omelets (page 98), warmed

1 slice sprouted grain bread (see page 33), toasted

¼ avocado (25g), smashed

¼ teaspoon everything bagel seasoning

Pinch of sprouts of your choice (arugula sprouts are my favorite)

1. In a small bowl, combine the maple syrup, lemon juice, and Dijon. Whisk to combine until smooth.

2. Arrange the greens on a large plate and drizzle with the dressing. Toss to combine, then lay the omelets over the greens.

3. Spread the toast with the avocado and sprinkle with the everything bagel seasoning. Top with the sprouts and enjoy alongside the greens and omelets.

NOTE: If using leftover Garden Vegetable Chickpea Omelets, you can warm them in the microwave for 30 to 40 seconds.

NUTRITION FACTS

FOR 1 SERVING: CALORIES: 297   PROTEIN: 15g   CARBS: 37g   FAT: 7g

"Egg" and Avocado Breakfast Sandwich

MAKES
1
SANDWICH

For this recipe, I took my favorite hearty, savory breakfast ingredients and piled them into one delicious sandwich. With rich, creamy avocado and hummus, it always hits the spot, and yet, thanks to plenty of greens, it never feels too heavy for the first meal of the day.

Spread the mustard over one slice of bread and the hummus over the other. Atop the hummus, layer the omelet, greens, avocado, and sprouts (if using). Drizzle with hot sauce, salsa, or tzatziki and top with the second slice of bread.

1 tablespoon coarse-ground Dijon mustard

2 slices of sprouted whole-grain bread (see page 33)

2 tablespoons hummus

1 Garden Vegetable Chickpea Omelet (page 98)

1 cup greens of your choice (I love arugula for this)

½ small avocado (50g), sliced

Sprouts (optional)

Hot sauce, salsa, or ¼ cup Tzatziki Sauce (page 221 or store-bought)

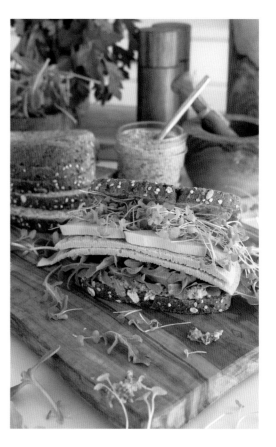

NUTRITION FACTS

FOR 1 SANDWICH: CALORIES: 377   PROTEIN: 16g   CARBS: 39g   FAT: 10g

Breakfast Tacos

SERVES
1
MAKES 3 TACOS

I love tacos. Morning, afternoon, or evening, rain or shine, if there's a meal to be had, there's a very good chance that it's going to be a taco for me. These check all the boxes—hearty, filling, flavorful, and delicious for any meal. But turning to my Garden Vegetable Chickpea Omelets here makes them feel extra breakfast-y. It's a great way to use up any leftovers, or you can do what I do and double or triple your batch of omelets to store in the refrigerator. Another tip: Try these with a drizzle of sugar-free maple syrup (I've listed my favorite on page 33). The salty-sweet effect is similar to letting your eggs and hash browns mingle with the maple syrup on your pancake plate.

Cooking spray (see page 33)

1 small Yukon Gold potato (154g), shredded

½ cup diced red bell pepper

¼ cup diced yellow onion

Garlic salt, to taste

1 Garden Vegetable Chickpea Omelet (page 98), chopped

3 (6-inch) corn tortillas

½ cup Pico de Gallo (page 208), or salsa of your choice

¼ small avocado (25g), peeled, pitted, and thinly sliced

---

1. Heat a medium nonstick skillet over medium-high heat. Lightly coat the pan with cooking spray and add the potato, pepper, and onion. Season with a pinch of garlic salt and sauté until the vegetables begin to brown and the potatoes are cooked through, 3 to 5 minutes. Add the chopped Garden Vegetable Chickpea Omelet to the pan and cook until it's heated through, about 1 minute.

2. Divide the vegetable and omelet mixture among the tortillas, top with the Pico de Gallo and avocado, and enjoy.

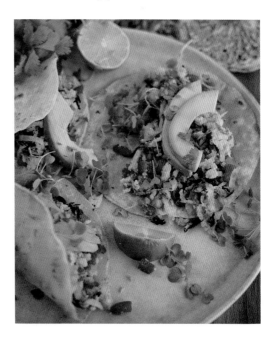

NUTRITION FACTS

FOR 1 SERVING: **CALORIES:** 435 **PROTEIN:** 13g **CARBS:** 70g **FAT:** 7.5g

CHAPTER 8

Lunch and Dinner

My recipes are designed around the Plantifully Simple mission of eating more and feeling better: They enable you to create meals that are full of fiber-rich, low-calorie-density ingredients. I also want to set you up to succeed, which means giving you ideas for dishes that will keep you satisfied between meals, especially at midday and in the evening when all you want to do is dive headfirst into something filling and delicious.

This chapter is the perfect marriage of those goals (if I do say so myself) and is stuffed with options for bowls, salads, wraps, sandwiches, and a variety of dishes that not only provide nutrition and sustenance but also deliver enough flavor and variety to scratch every itch and suit every mood. Best of all, I think you'll be amazed at just how much you can eat, and that you'll delight in seeing how many of your favorite dishes can be made low-fat and low-calorie with a few simple swaps.

Sweet Potato Black Bean Curry

SERVES
1

This curry is one of my favorite ways to enjoy sweet potatoes because they balance the otherwise deeply savory flavors of this dish. It's especially cozy and fortifying on a chilly fall or winter day thanks to hearty black beans and plenty of kale. I love how the vegetables become tender and aromatic after simmering in a coconut milk broth, which gets a punch of flavor and a sunny glow from yellow curry paste (aka the easiest way to transform a dish with barely any work), plus bright pops of flavor from cilantro and lime. When poured over steamed rice, it's a deeply comforting yet light-feeling dish that warms and fills the belly.

1 medium sweet potato (250g)

¼ cup diced yellow onion

1 cup unsweetened almond milk

¾ cup canned light coconut milk

3 teaspoons yellow curry paste, plus more to taste

2 cups chopped kale leaves (see Note on page 86)

¼ cup canned black beans, drained and rinsed

1 teaspoon fresh lime juice

½ teaspoon sea salt, plus more to taste

Stevia or maple syrup, to taste

½ cup packed fresh cilantro, chopped

1 cup steamed white rice, for serving

1. Preheat the oven to 425°F. Line a baking sheet with parchment paper.

2. Use a fork to pierce the sweet potato all over. Place the potato on the prepared baking sheet and bake for 40 minutes or until a knife easily slides in. Allow the potato to cool slightly, then use your hands to remove and discard the skin. Cut the potato into bite-size cubes. Set aside.

3. In a medium pot over medium-high heat, sauté the onions until they begin to brown, about 3 minutes. Add the almond milk, coconut milk, and curry paste and stir until the curry paste is completely incorporated.

4. Add the kale, beans, lime juice, and salt and cook, stirring, until the kale has wilted and everything is heated through, about 5 minutes. Season with a couple of drops of Stevia and/or more salt, if needed. Stir in the cilantro and serve over rice.

NUTRITION FACTS (includes sweetening with Stevia)
FOR 1 SERVING: CALORIES: 623 PROTEIN: 15g CARBS: 93g FAT: 14g

Lemon Chickpea Soup

SERVES
1

This is the perfect recipe for those nights when you barely have enough energy to finish your day strong but don't have anything prepped. Chickpeas are one of the greatest tools in your plant-based cooking tool box, because you can just grab them from your pantry; they're extremely nutrient-dense and have a ton of fiber and protein; and they take on just about any flavor you add to them. I love combining these legumes with a bright, lemony broth and wilted kale for a soup that's simple, light, and deeply nourishing.

In a medium pot over medium heat, combine the chickpeas, onion, bouillon cubes, garlic, lemon juice, and oregano. Stir in the water and bring the mixture to a simmer. Cook for 10 minutes, until the soup is heated through and the flavors have melded. Turn off the heat, add the kale, and allow it to wilt, about 2 minutes. Stir in the milk and season with the garlic salt and pepper to taste. Garnish with the parsley and serve.

1 (15-ounce) can chickpeas, drained and rinsed

½ small yellow onion (110g), diced

2 vegan bouillon cubes
(see page 33), plus more to taste

1 tablespoon minced garlic

Juice of 1 lemon

1 teaspoon dried oregano

4 cups water

1½ cups chopped kale leaves
(see Note on page 186)

1 cup plain, unsweetened plant-
based milk

Garlic salt, to taste

Freshly ground black pepper, to taste

Chopped fresh parsley, for garnish

NUTRITION FACTS

FOR 1 RECIPE: CALORIES: 474   PROTEIN: 21g   CARBS: 46g   FAT: 16g

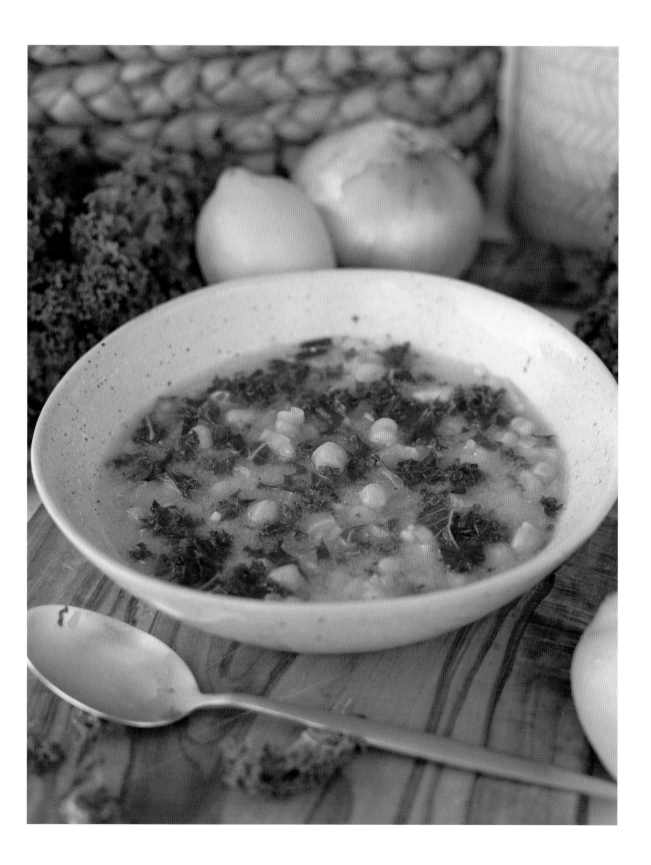

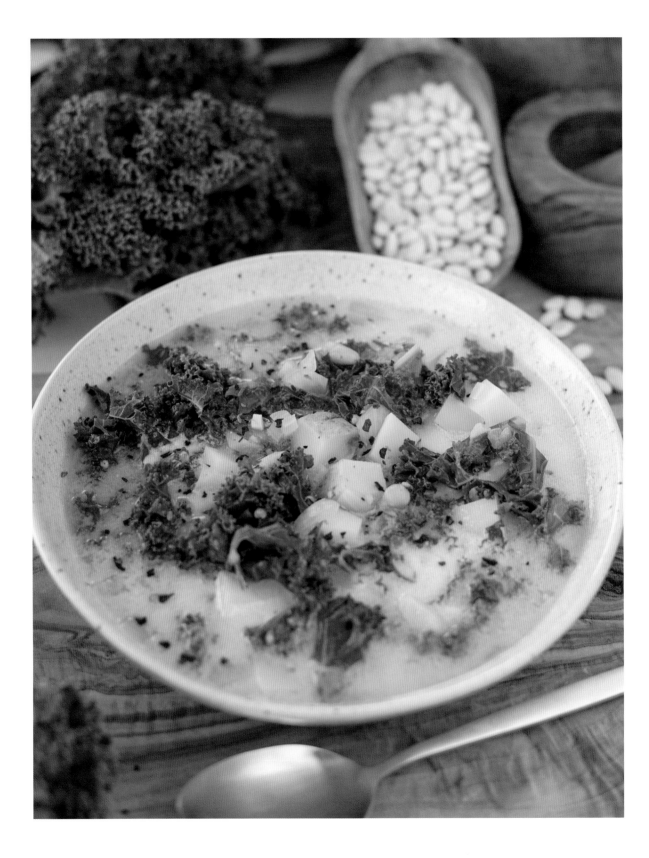

Potato Kale Soup

SERVES
2
MAKES 8 CUPS

When I was growing up, my mom and I would have weekly mother-daughter date nights at Olive Garden, and almost every single time, I ordered the Zuppa Toscana. It was rich and creamy and loaded with vegetables and spicy Italian sausage. At the time, it was nothing short of perfection. Now, whenever I crave that familiar flavor and the comfort that comes with it, I reach for this recipe. Thanks to a few simple swaps—plant-based milk for cream, white beans and potatoes for heartiness instead of sausage, heaps of nutrient-rich kale—I can enjoy it whenever I want and feel really good about it.

Cooking spray (see page 33)
1 medium yellow onion
1 tablespoon minced garlic
1 large Yukon gold potato (400g), diced
1 (15-ounce) can (245g) white beans, drained and rinsed
2 vegan bouillon cubes (see page 33)
6 cups water
1 bunch of kale leaves (120g), chopped (6 cups)
1 cup plain, unsweetened almond milk
1 teaspoon chili flakes
1½ teaspoon garlic salt, or more to taste

1. Heat a medium pot over medium heat. If you like, you can coat it with cooking spray to encourage even cooking, but it isn't necessary. Add the onion and cook until softened, 3 to 4 minutes. If it starts to stick, you can add a splash of water. Add the garlic and cook for 1 minute, just until fragrant and not yet beginning to brown. Add the potato, white beans, and bouillon cubes, then stir in the water.

2. Bring the mixture to a boil, uncovered, and boil for 15 minutes, until the potatoes are fork tender. Turn off the heat and stir in the kale and almond milk. Allow the kale to wilt for a few minutes, then add the chili flakes and season to taste with garlic salt.

> NOTE: Each serving is so hearty (4 cups) because it's a relatively light soup, and this will ensure that you're getting enough calories and sustenance to tide you over until your next meal.

NUTRITION FACTS
FOR 4 CUPS: **CALORIES:** 436g **PROTEIN:** 20g **CARBS:** 62g **FAT:** 6g

Lentil Mushroom Stew

Maybe it's because I live in Colorado and love spending time outside in the snow, but a bowl of warm, comforting soup is one of my favorite meals. This recipe gets a satisfying "meatiness" from mushrooms, plus belly-filling lentils and potatoes that soak up all the delicious flavor from a garlic-and-oregano-scented broth made creamy with almond milk. I love making this in an Instant Pot because of how fast and hands-off it is, but even on the stovetop it comes together in barely any time.

Cooking spray (page 33, optional)

16 ounces baby bella mushrooms, wiped clean and quartered

1 medium yellow onion, chopped

1 cup peeled and diced carrots (3 medium carrots)

3 garlic cloves, minced

2 medium russet or Yukon Gold potatoes (426g), cut into 1-inch pieces

1 (14-ounce) can or jar tomato sauce

1 cup dry brown lentils (208g; see Note)

3 vegan bouillon cubes (see page 33)

1 dried bay leaf

1 teaspoon sea salt

½ teaspoon dried oregano

Freshly ground black pepper, to taste

3 cups water

1 cup plain, unsweetened almond milk

Fresh parsley, chopped, to garnish

1. **If using an Instant Pot:** Set the pot to the Sauté setting and add the mushrooms, onion, carrots, and garlic. Cook the vegetables, stirring occasionally, until they're tender, 5 to 8 minutes.

2. Add the potatoes, tomato sauce, lentils, bouillon cubes, bay leaf, salt, oregano, and a couple of twists of pepper. Stir in the water. Secure the lid and cook on the high pressure setting for 15 minutes, then allow the pressure to release naturally. (This typically takes about 40 minutes total.)

3. Remove the lid, discard the bay leaf, and stir in the almond milk. Adjust the seasonings to taste, if needed, and garnish with the parsley.

4. **If making on the stovetop:** Heat a medium or large saucepan over medium-high heat. If you like, you can coat it with cooking spray to encourage even cooking, but it isn't necessary. Add the mushrooms, onion, carrots, and garlic and sauté, stirring occasionally, until the vegetables are soft, 5 to 8 minutes. If the vegetables start to stick, you can add a splash of water.

5. Add the potatoes, tomato sauce, lentils, bouillon cubes, bay leaf, salt, oregano, and a couple of twists of pepper. Stir in the water and bring the mixture to a simmer. Cook, covered and stirring occasionally, for 15 to 20 minutes, or until the potatoes are tender.

NOTE: If making this on the stovetop, substitute 2 (14-ounce) cans of lentils, drained, for the dried ones.

6. Remove and discard the bay leaf and stir in the almond milk. Adjust the seasonings to taste, and serve garnished with the chopped parsley.

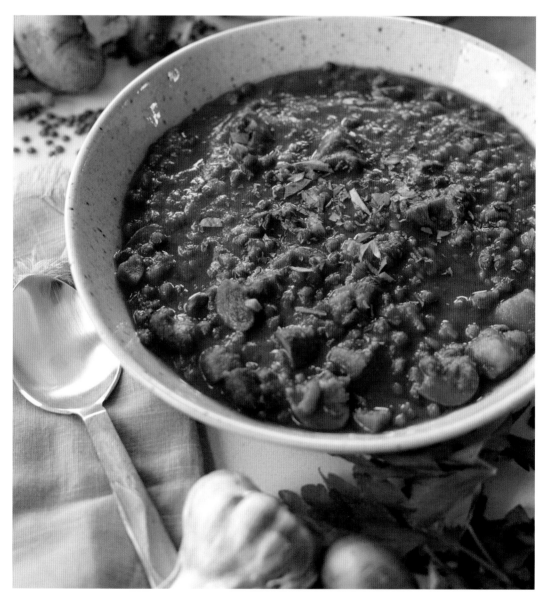

NUTRITION FACTS
FOR 1 SERVING (2 CUPS): **CALORIES:** 384 **PROTEIN:** 22g **CARBS:** 55g **FAT:** 4g

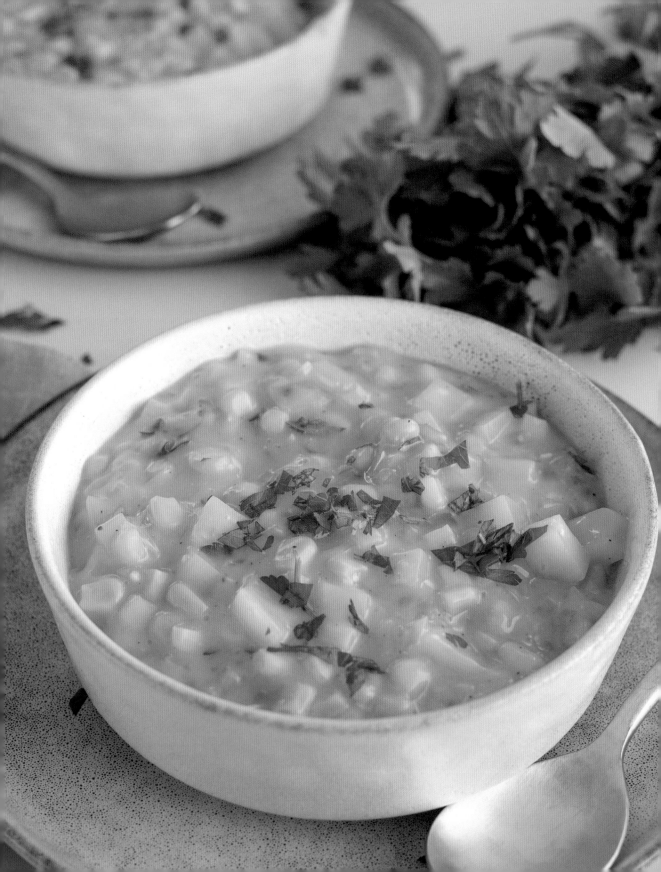

Potato Corn Chowder

SERVES
2
MAKES 5 CUPS

I couldn't promise a book full of recipes that would help you embrace plant-based eating and never look back and not include the creamiest, dreamiest chowder ever. This rich, thick soup is loaded with buttery potatoes and sweet pops of corn and is as simple to make as it is warming and filling. This dish is perfect for a chilly day, but I also like to make it at the beginning of the week and have it on hand as an easy meal. It will keep in the refrigerator for up to 5 days.

1 medium yellow onion, chopped

½ cup chopped celery (about 2 medium stalks)

3 garlic cloves, minced

2 medium to large russet potatoes (455g), peeled and diced

3 vegan bouillon cubes (see page 33)

3 cups water

1 cup plain, unsweetened almond milk

¼ cup cornstarch

1 (15-ounce) can corn kernels, drained, or 1¼ cups fresh or frozen corn kernels

¼ cup chopped fresh parsley leaves, for serving

Sea salt and freshly ground black pepper, to taste

1. In a medium or large pot, combine the onion and celery. Sauté over medium-high heat until the onions begin to soften, 3 to 4 minutes. Add the garlic and cook until fragrant and just beginning to soften, about 1 minute.

2. Add the potatoes, bouillon cubes, and water and bring to a boil. Reduce to a simmer and cook, uncovered and stirring occasionally, until the potatoes are fork tender, about 15 minutes.

3. Meanwhile, in a small bowl, whisk together the almond milk and cornstarch to make a slurry. When the potatoes are tender, add the almond milk slurry and the corn to the soup. Increase the heat to medium-high to bring to a boil and cook for 1 minute. The soup should have a gravy-like consistency.

4. Remove the pot from the heat, stir in the parsley, and season with salt and pepper as desired. Serve warm.

NUTRITION FACTS

FOR 1 SERVING (2½ CUPS): CALORIES: 405 PROTEIN: 10g CARBS: 75g FAT: 7g

Everything Bagel Wrap

SERVES

1

Everything bagels are one of my obsessions, so I was determined to come up with a recipe that would bring me their flavor and texture without the belly-bomb feeling of an actual bagel. This wrap uses lavash, which is a soft, chewy flatbread, and I spread it with Everything Bagel Bean Dip and then load it with veggies. This is my way of scratching that everything bagel craving whenever I want, without spiking my glucose and leaving me hungry an hour later the way a bagel will. This wrap also makes a great cold lunch option and packs nicely, especially for a picnic or a hike.

½ cup **Everything Bagel Bean Dip** (page 205)

1 **lavash bread wrap** (see page 34)

½ medium **bell pepper**, seeded and sliced

1 medium **carrot**, shredded

¼ cup sliced **red onion**

1 medium **tomato**, sliced

½ medium **avocado** (50g), peeled, pitted, and sliced

6 **butter lettuce leaves** (or lettuce of your choice)

Spread the dip evenly over the lavash. Layer on the bell pepper, carrot, onion, tomato, avocado, and lettuce. Roll up the wrap and enjoy.

NUTRITION FACTS
FOR ONE WRAP: CALORIES: 444   PROTEIN: 24g   CARBS: 44g   FAT: 12g

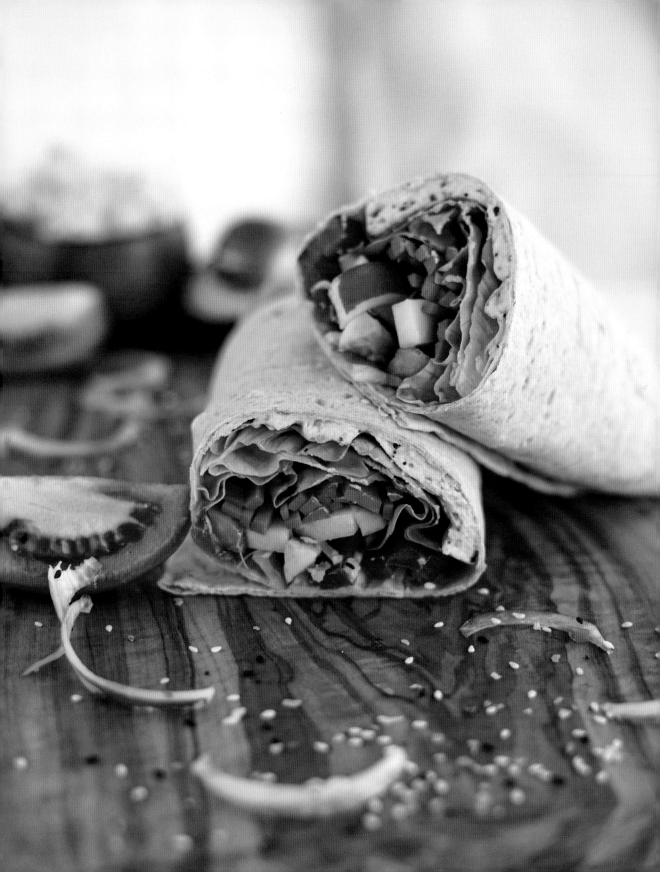

Falafel Cauliflower Pitas

SERVES
1
MAKES 3 PITAS

As far as plant-based treats go, falafel is probably at the top of my list. There's really nothing like
a crispy ball of spiced and fried chickpeas stuffed
into a pita and topped with creamy tzatziki and all
the fresh veggies. When I was looking for a healthier way to enjoy these classic flavors but without
the deep frying, I figured out that when you season
cauliflower with the same seasonings and roast it
until golden and crisp, it's an extremely satisfying
stand-in for the falafel but with much more nutrition and much less oil.

---

4 cups cauliflower florets, cut into bite-size pieces

Juice of ½ lemon

1 teaspoon ground coriander

¾ teaspoon garlic salt

½ teaspoon ground cumin

¼ teaspoon chili powder (optional)

¼ teaspoon ground turmeric

¼ teaspoon freshly ground black pepper

Pinch of ground cinnamon

Cooking spray (see page 33)

3 low-calorie pitas (see page 34)

**1 cup spring greens or chopped
romaine, Bibb, or butter lettuce**

1 medium Roma tomato, sliced

½ small cucumber, sliced

¼ cup sliced red onion

½ cup Tzatziki Sauce (page 221)

1 tablespoon chopped fresh parsley leaves

1 tablespoon chopped fresh cilantro leaves

---

1. Preheat the oven to 425°F. Line a baking sheet
    with parchment paper and set aside.

2. In a large bowl, combine the cauliflower, lemon
    juice, coriander, garlic salt, cumin, chili powder
    (if using), turmeric, pepper, and cinnamon. Toss
    to coat the cauliflower well.

3. Transfer the mixture to the prepared baking
    sheet and spread it in a single, even layer. Lightly
    coat with cooking spray, which will help the
    cauliflower crisp up as it roasts. Roast for 20
    to 25 minutes, until the cauliflower begins to
    brown. Remove from the oven and allow the
    cauliflower to cool slightly.

4. Divide the cauliflower between the three pitas
    and layer with the greens, tomato, cucumber,
    and onion. Top each pita with ¼ cup of Tzatziki
    Sauce and garnish with the parsley and cilantro.

NUTRITION FACTS
FOR 1 SERVING: CALORIES: 405   PROTEIN: 29g   CARBS: 44g   FAT: 9g

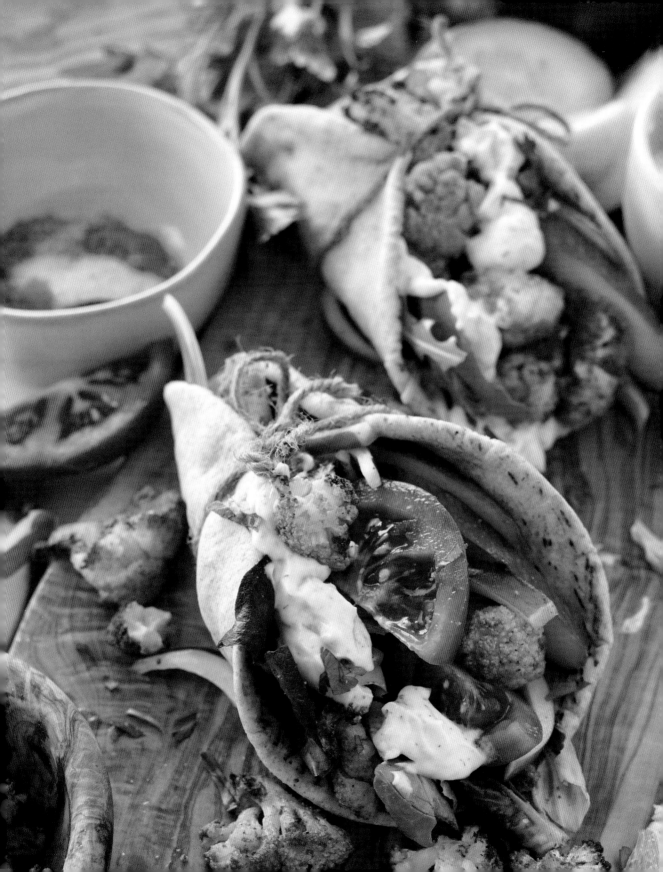

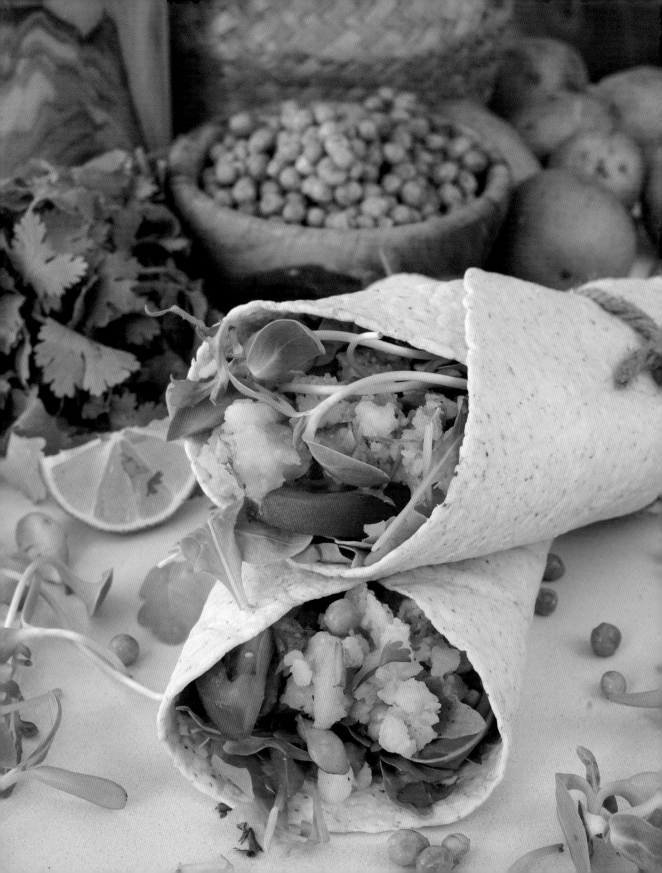

Samosa Wraps

Indian samosas, or fried bundles of spiced mashed potato, are one of my favorite foods—but they're also high in fat and calories. I wanted to come up with a version that still delivers all that flavor and texture but in a way that works for you if you're keeping an eye on calorie density. The trick is to swap out the deep fryer for the oven, use low-calorie wraps, and add a side of greens.

1 large Yukon Gold potato (330g)
¼ cup fresh or frozen peas
1 tablespoon chopped fresh cilantro leaves
1 teaspoon fresh lime juice
½ teaspoon curry powder
½ teaspoon garlic powder
¼ teaspoon onion powder
¼ teaspoon sea salt
2 low-calorie wraps (see page 37)
1 medium Roma tomato, sliced
4 cups greens (I like arugula for this)

1. Preheat the oven to 425°F. Pierce the potato all over and bake on a baking sheet for 45 minutes, until fork tender.

2. Allow the potato to cool slightly while you cook the peas. In a small or medium pot, bring a couple of inches of water to a simmer over medium heat. Add the peas and boil until bright green and tender, about 30 seconds. Transfer the peas to a bowl and set aside.

3. Transfer the potato to a medium bowl and use a fork or potato masher to mash until smooth. Add the peas, cilantro, lime juice, curry powder, garlic powder, onion powder, and salt and mix well to combine.

4. Divide the potato mixture between the two wraps. Top with the tomato and greens, roll up the wraps, and enjoy!

NUTRITION FACTS
FOR 1 SERVING: CALORIES: 489   PROTEIN: 28g   CARBS: 75g   FAT: 5g

Herby White Bean Sammy

I can't decide what I love more about this sandwich—that it's packed with protein and other essential nutrients, or that the combination of the Herby Bean Dip and Smokehouse Ranch is creamy, filling, and flavorful and makes this taste like your favorite mayo-based salad. And then there's the fact that you can have a batch of the spread and dressing ready to go in the fridge for whenever you need a meal quickly. I especially love this sandwich packed up for road trips, hikes, or picnics.

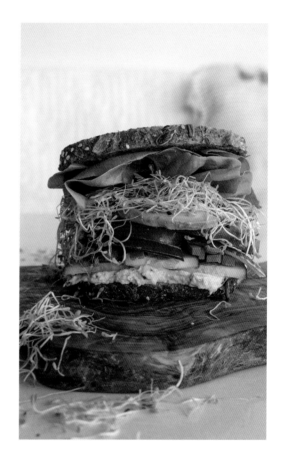

---

2 slices sprouted whole-grain bread
(see page 33), toasted

½ cup Herby Bean Dip (page 206)

2 tablespoons Smokehouse Ranch (page 197)

1 medium carrot, shredded

1 small tomato, sliced

½ small cucumber, sliced

¼ medium avocado (25g), peeled, pitted, and sliced

¼ cup sliced red onion

¼ cup sprouts of your choice

2 lettuce leaves of your choice

Spread one slice of the toasted bread with the Herby Bean Dip and drizzle the Smokehouse Ranch over it. Top with the carrot, tomato, cucumber, avocado, onion, sprouts, and lettuce leaves and the second slice of bread.

NOTE: The Herby Bean Dip also makes a great snack paired with a low-calorie pita (see page 34).

NUTRITION FACTS

FOR 1 SERVING: **CALORIES:** 465 **PROTEIN:** 23g **CARBS:** 56g **FAT:** 10g

Apple Pimento Grilled Cheese with Caramelized Onions and Arugula

SERVES
2
MAKES 2 SANDWICHES

I think we can all agree that grilled cheese is the universal comfort food, and the thought of having to leave behind an ooey, gooey sandwich that reminds you of your favorite childhood meal when transitioning to a plant-based diet can be difficult. I don't believe in ever feeling deprived or not having the option to enjoy decadent-feeling foods, and therefore I developed this "gourmet" version of the classic. Caramelized onions bring a savory sweetness to my Pimento Cheese Sauce, while apple slices and arugula lend a pop of tart crunch and peppery freshness.

---

1 small sweet yellow onion, sliced
⅛ teaspoon garlic salt
4 slices sprouted whole-grain bread (see page 33)
½ cup Pimento Cheese Sauce (page 225)
1 small Honeycrisp apple, cored and sliced
1 cup arugula

---

1. Add the onions to a medium or large non-stick pan and season with the garlic salt. Over medium-high heat, allow the onions to brown on one side undisturbed, 2 to 3 minutes. Give them a stir and leave them to brown once again for another 2 to 3 minutes, until soft and golden. Transfer the onions to a plate and wipe out the pan.

2. Spread each slice of bread with ¼ cup of the Pimento Cheese Sauce. Top each slice with half of the apple slices, caramelized onions, and arugula. Top each sandwich with the second slice of bread.

3. In the same pan you used for the onions, over medium heat or on a griddle, toast the first sandwich until the bottom slice of bread is golden brown, about 2 minutes. Carefully flip the sandwich—a silicone spatula works well here—and cook for another 2 minutes or until browned on the other side.

4. Transfer to a plate and repeat with the second sandwich. Enjoy warm.

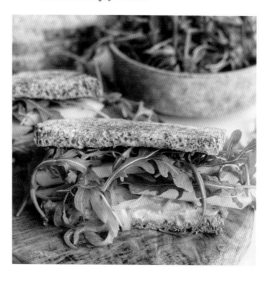

NUTRITION FACTS
FOR 1 SERVING: **CALORIES:** 474 **PROTEIN:** 19g **CARBS:** 74g **FAT:** 5g

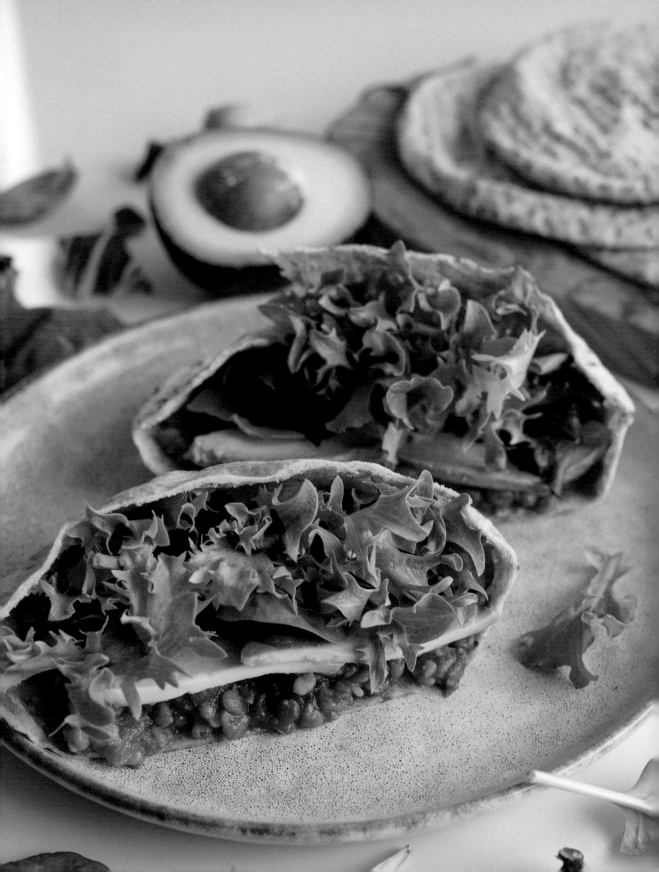

Sloppy Joe Pockets

SERVES
2
MAKES 2
SANDWICHES

One of my favorite dinners when I was growing up was Sloppy Joe night. I couldn't get enough of the sweet, spiced, saucy, meaty filling heaped onto a bun. So I was excited when I finally nailed this recipe. When you simmer hearty lentils and mushrooms in a tomato-y sauce spiked with smoked paprika and maple syrup and then stuff them into a pita with some avocado, you get the exact same effect but with a fraction of the calories. This is a major crowd pleaser.

½ cup diced white or baby bella mushrooms (optional; see Note)

¼ cup diced yellow onion

1 tablespoon water

1 (15-ounce) can brown lentils (1½ cups), drained and rinsed

¼ cup tomato sauce

¼ cup ketchup

¼ cup diced red bell pepper

¼ teaspoon garlic powder

¼ teaspoon smoked paprika

¼ teaspoon sea salt

2 tablespoons maple syrup or stevia

1 low-calorie pita (see page 34)

1 cup greens of your choice

¼ medium avocado (25g), peeled, pitted, and sliced (optional)

---

1. In a medium saucepan, combine the mushrooms, if using, and onion with the water. Sauté over medium-high heat until the onions are soft, about 3 minutes. Add the lentils, tomato sauce, ketchup, bell pepper, garlic powder, smoked paprika, and salt and simmer, stirring occasionally, for 5 minutes. You want the mixture to be warmed through and the flavors to have melded. Add the maple syrup or stevia and adjust any of the seasonings as desired.

2. Slice the pita in half. Divide the lentil mixture between the pita pockets, then add the greens and avocado, if desired.

> **NOTE:** You don't have to use the mushrooms, but they add even more volume and nutrition to the meal.

NUTRITION FACTS
FOR 1 PITA WITH LENTIL FILLING AND AVOCADO: CALORIES: 651 **PROTEIN:** 36g **CARBS:** 98g **FAT:** 7g

Apple Chickpea Salad Sandwich

SERVES
4
MAKES 4
SANDWICHES

My mom always made the most amazing chicken salad, so when I switched to a plant-based diet, I knew I would need to come up with a version I could have whenever I missed that dish—which is pretty much all the time. Chickpeas are a great chicken substitute here because of their substantial texture, mild flavor, and high protein content. When combined with my mom's signature mix of sweet and savory ingredients (bits of crunchy apple are a game-changer!), you get a light and flavorful salad that's perfect for heaping on bread.

1 (15-ounce) can chickpeas, drained and rinsed

½ cup plain, unsweetened coconut yogurt (see page 34)

½ cup diced Fuji apple

⅓ cup finely diced celery

⅓ cup finely diced red onion

1 teaspoon fresh lemon juice

½ teaspoon garlic salt

3 drops of stevia or monk fruit sweetener

Freshly ground black pepper, to taste

8 slices sprouted whole-grain bread (see page 33)

8 romaine lettuce leaves

1 cup sprouts

1. In a medium bowl, use a fork or potato masher to mash the chickpeas. (They'll be a little chunky, and that's okay!) Add the yogurt, apple, celery, onion, lemon juice, garlic salt, stevia, and a few twists of black pepper. Mix well to combine.

2. Top 4 slices of the bread with ½ cup of the filling each. Add two lettuce leaves to each sandwich, followed by ¼ cup of the sprouts. Top each sandwich with the second slice of bread and serve.

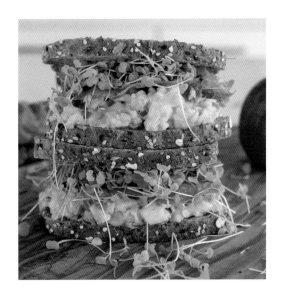

NOTE: If you're not serving four sandwiches at once, this salad will keep in the fridge for up to 3 days.

NUTRITION FACTS

FOR 1 SANDWICH: CALORIES: 286   PROTEIN: 14g   CARBS: 39g   FAT: 4g

Saucy Portobello Sammies

MAKES
1
SANDWICH

Give me two slices of bread, a stack of veggies, and some saucy condiments, and I'm a happy girl. But this recipe's particular combination of mushrooms smothered in sweet barbecue sauce and draped in homemade ranch dressing is seriously next level. It tastes like the kind of deluxe sandwich you could get at a bar and grill, but as you can probably guess, I've given it a low-calorie, low-fat makeover.

Cooking spray (see page 33, optional)

8 ounces portobello mushrooms, wiped clean, stems removed, and sliced

2 tablespoons of your favorite barbecue sauce (ideally one around 70 calories or fewer for 2 tablespoons)

2 slices sprouted whole-grain bread (see page 33)

2 tablespoons Smokehouse Ranch (page 197)

2 slices red onion

1 cup spring greens

½ cup alfalfa sprouts

1. Heat a large nonstick skillet over medium-high heat. If you like, you can coat it with cooking spray to encourage the mushrooms to brown, but it isn't necessary. Add the sliced mushrooms and cook, stirring occasionally, until they soften and begin to brown, about 8 minutes. If the mushrooms begin to stick, you can add a splash of water. Remove the pan from the heat.

2. In a small bowl, combine the mushrooms with the barbecue sauce and toss to coat. Top 1 slice of bread with the mushrooms, then add the ranch, onion, greens, and sprouts. Top with the second slice of bread and enjoy.

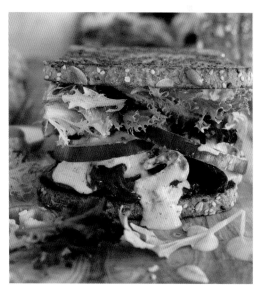

NUTRITION FACTS
FOR 1 SERVING (1 SANDWICH):   CALORIES: 322   PROTEIN: 13g   CARBS: 46g   FAT: 6g

Green Goddess Sammy

MAKES
1
SANDWICH

Sandwiches are a great cold lunch option, especially if you bring your lunch to work or need to pack for a road trip. For this recipe, which has become a major go-to for me, I combine white beans and avocado to create a creamy spread that I can load up with as many veggies as possible. I love all the flavor and fiber. You'll notice that I didn't include exact measures for the veggies; that's because these low-calorie additions won't make or break your daily calorie count but will keep you feeling full until your next meal. This is the time to go big!

½ **cup (80g) canned white beans,
drained and rinsed**

½ **medium avocado (50g)**

1 tablespoon fresh lemon juice

Garlic salt, to taste

**2 slices sprouted grain bread
(see page 33), toasted**

Your favorite hot sauce (optional)

Cucumber slices

Lettuce

Sprouts

---

1.   In a small bowl, use a fork to mash together the beans, avocado, and lemon juice. Season with garlic salt to taste.

2.   Spread the bean mash over one slice of bread, top with a dash of hot sauce (if desired), and heap high with cucumber, lettuce, and sprouts. Top with the remaining slice of bread and serve.

NUTRITION FACTS
FOR 1 SERVING (1 SANDWICH):   **CALORIES:** 385   **PROTEIN:** 20g   **CARBS:** 43g   **FAT:** 9g

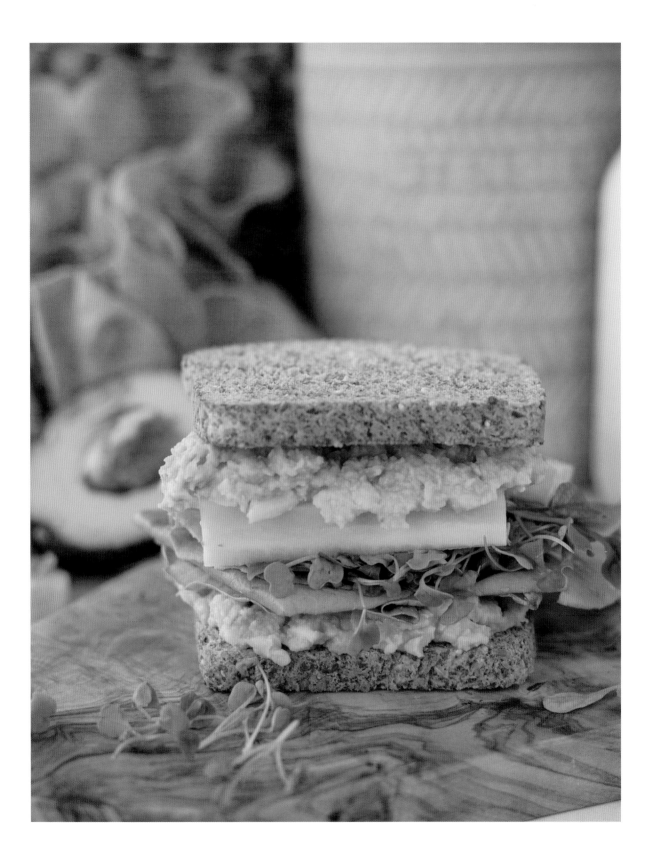

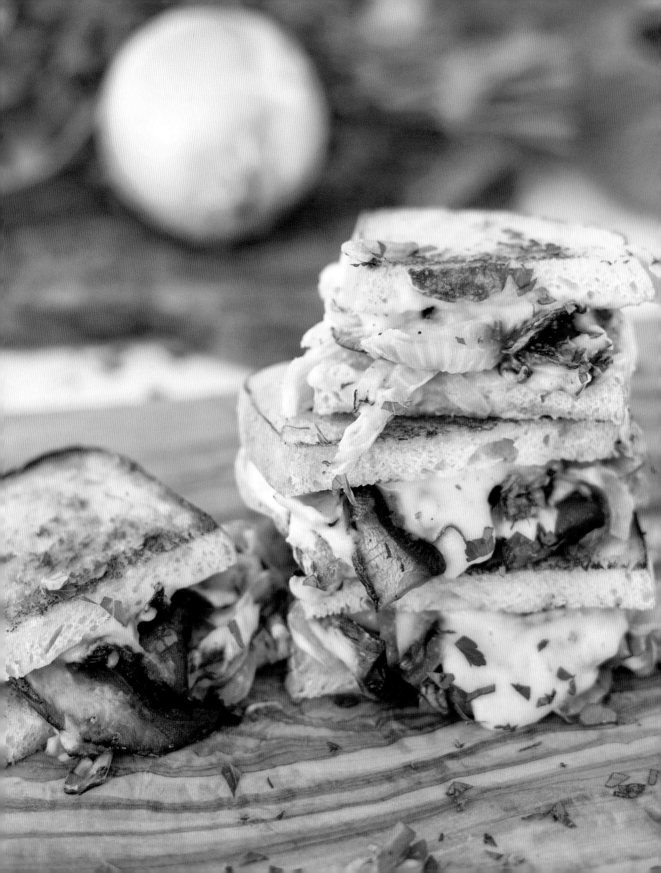

Grilled "Steak" and Cheese Sammy

MAKES
1
SANDWICH

This sandwich gives major Philly cheesesteak vibes, down to how many napkins you need to eat it! People barely notice that mushrooms are standing in for meat, because the selling points are all the caramelized onions and poblano-spiked cheese sauce that get piled on the top. You seriously won't believe how low in calories this actually is.

Cooking spray (see page 33, optional)

1 portobello mushroom cap (110g), wiped clean and thinly sliced

½ small yellow onion, thinly sliced

Garlic salt, to taste

½ cup Poblano Cheese Sauce (page 216), cold

2 slices of sprouted grain bread (see page 33)

---

1. Heat a large nonstick skillet over medium-high heat. If you like, you can coat it with cooking spray to encourage even cooking, but it isn't necessary. Add the mushroom and onion with a pinch of garlic salt and sauté until the vegetables have softened, about 8 minutes. If they start to stick, you can add a splash of water. Remove the pan from the heat.

2. Spread the Poblano Cheese Sauce over one slice of bread. Top the cheese with the mushroom and onion mixture, followed by the second slice of bread.

3. Wipe out your nonstick skillet, lightly coat it with cooking spray, and return it to medium heat. Add the sandwich and grill until golden brown on the first side, about 3 minutes. Carefully flip the sandwich and repeat on the other side. Serve warm.

NUTRITION FACTS
FOR 1 SERVING (1 SANDWICH):   CALORIES: 268   PROTEIN: 12g   CARBS: 38g   FAT: 5g

Black Bean Tacos
with Avocado Lime Crema

SERVES
1
MAKES 4
TACOS

I like to call these my "lazy girl tacos." On busy nights when I barely have enough energy to cook, I can just pull out some corn tortillas, a can of fat-free refried beans, and the jar of my Avocado Lime Crema that I usually keep stashed in the fridge for such emergencies, and dinner is served. That said, you don't need to wait until things are dire to make them! And don't be fooled by the simple ingredients—these tacos are packed with flavor from the layers of condiments.

¾ cup (195g) canned fat-free black refried beans

4 (6-inch) corn tortillas

Cooking spray (see page 33, optional)

3 tablespoons Avocado Lime Crema
(page 218; see Note)

Your favorite hot sauce (optional)

¼ cup Pimento Cheese Sauce
(page 225), warmed (optional)

---

1. Spread the beans over half of each tortilla. Set aside.

2. Heat a nonstick pan over medium-high heat. If you like, you can coat it with cooking spray to encourage even cooking, but it isn't necessary.

3. Fold each tortilla in half and add them to the pan. Cook until the first side is golden brown, about 3 minutes, then flip and repeat on the other side.

4. Transfer the tacos to a plate and top with the Avocado Lime Crema, hot sauce, and/or Pimento Cheese Sauce.

NOTE: If you don't have Avocado Lime Crema handy and can't be bothered to whip up a batch (I get it!), simply top these with a few thin slices (25g) of avocado and a squeeze of lime juice.

If you want to add a little more kick to the beans, stir in 2 to 3 tablespoons of chopped pickled jalapeños.

NUTRITION FACTS

FOR 1 SERVING (4 TACOS):   CALORIES: 427   PROTEIN: 16g   CARBS: 60g   FAT: 8g

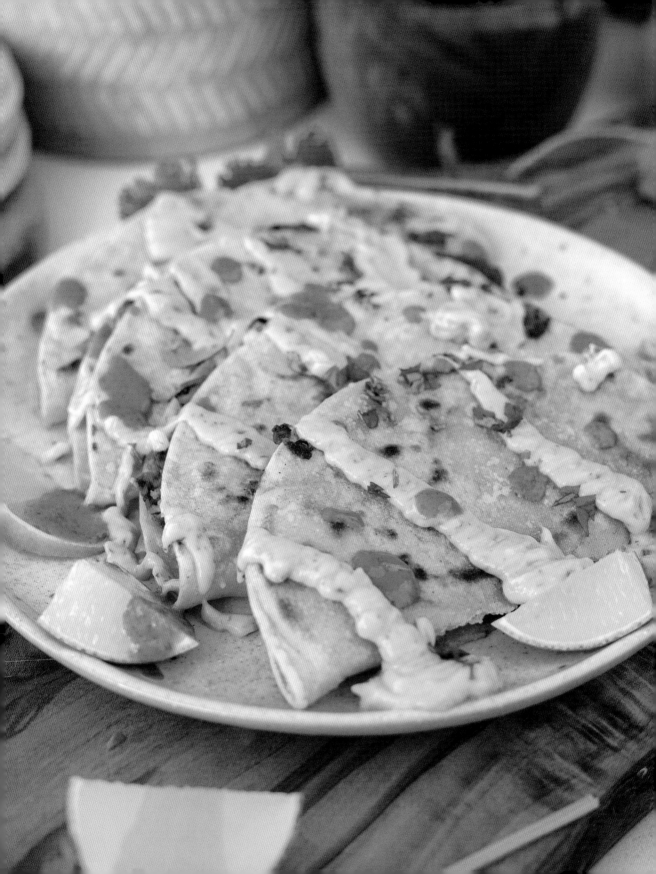

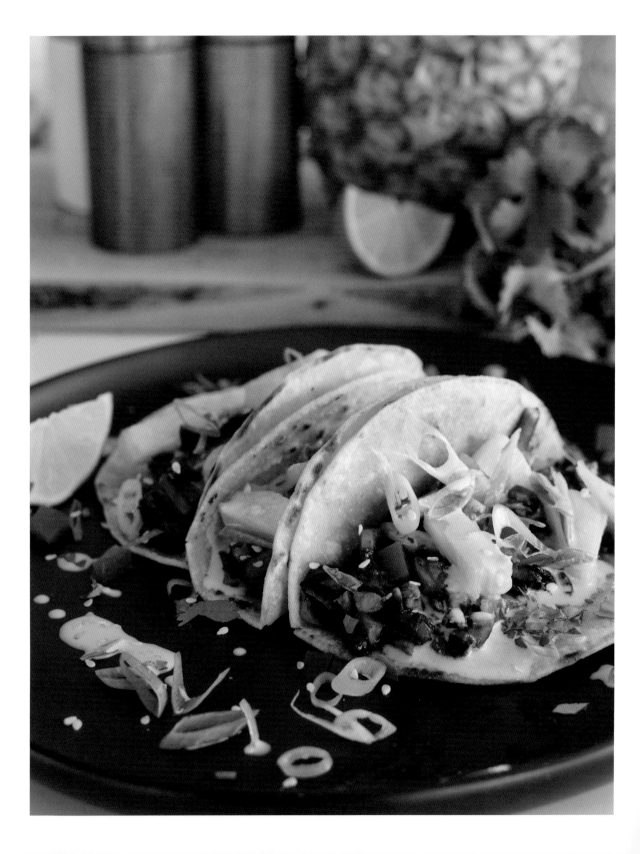

Hawaiian Street Cart Tacos

Tacos aren't just for Tuesdays in my house. I could eat them every night—especially these, which are a mash-up of flavors that I fell in love with in Hawaii. The tanginess of the barbecue sauce mixed with the sweet pineapple and rounded out with my Smokehouse Ranch is absolutely crave-worthy, especially when it's layered with meaty portobello mushrooms.

Cooking spray (see page 33, optional)

8 ounces portobello mushrooms, wiped clean, stems removed, and chopped

¼ teaspoon garlic salt

2 tablespoons of your favorite sweet barbecue sauce (I like Sweet Baby Ray's)

4 (6-inch) corn tortillas

½ cup diced canned or fresh pineapple (see Note on page 171)

¼ cup diced red bell pepper

1 scallion, sliced (white and green parts)

Lime, for serving

2 tablespoons Smokehouse Ranch (page 197)

Chopped fresh cilantro leaves, for garnish

---

1. Heat a large nonstick pan over medium-high heat. If you like, you can coat it with cooking spray to encourage even cooking, but it isn't necessary. Add the mushrooms and season with the garlic salt. Cook until the mushrooms soften and begin to brown, 5 to 8 minutes. If they start to stick, you can add a splash of water. Transfer the mushrooms to a small bowl and toss them with the barbecue sauce. Set aside.

2. Wipe out the pan and lightly coat it with cooking spray. Place the pan over medium heat and, one at a time, warm the tortillas just enough to cook off the raw corn flavor and lightly brown on both sides, 1 to 2 minutes per side.

3. Divide the mushroom filling among the tortillas. Top with the pineapple, bell pepper, and scallion. Add a squeeze of lime, then drizzle the Smokehouse Ranch over the top. Sprinkle with cilantro and serve.

NUTRITION FACTS
FOR 1 SERVING (4 TACOS), INCLUDING DRESSING: CALORIES: 372   PROTEIN: 9g   CARBS: 69g   FAT: 4g

Food Truck Tacos

SERVES
1
MAKES 4
TACOS

Mushrooms are one of my favorite plant-based substitutions for meat. Their texture is dense and chewy, and their savory, earthy flavor is delicious on its own but also pairs well with just about any seasoning or sauce. So, when I'm in the mood for a taco I can really sink my teeth into—which is often—I reach for mushrooms that I've tossed with smoky paprika and a Mexican seasoning blend. Topped off with tomato, onion, and avocado, these tacos rival those you'd get at any food truck, any day.

Cooking spray (see page 33)

8 ounces portobello mushrooms, wiped clean, stemmed, and chopped

1 teaspoon smoked paprika

1 teaspoon Mexican seasoning blend (I like Frontier's Mexican Fiesta Seasoning)

¼ teaspoon garlic salt

4 (6-inch) corn tortillas

1 Roma tomato, diced

¼ cup diced red onion

½ small avocado (50g)

Lime, for serving

Chopped fresh cilantro, for serving

---

1. Heat a large nonstick skillet over medium-high heat. If you like, you can coat it with cooking spray to encourage the mushrooms to brown, but it isn't necessary. Add the mushrooms and season with the paprika, Mexican seasoning blend, and garlic salt. Cook until the mushrooms soften and begin to brown, 5 to 8 minutes. If they start to stick, you can add a splash of water. Transfer the mushrooms to a small bowl and set aside.

2. Wipe out the pan and lightly coat it with cooking spray. Place the pan over medium heat and, one at a time, warm the tortillas just enough to cook off the raw corn flavor and lightly brown on both sides, 1 to 2 minutes per side.

3. Divide the mushrooms between the tortillas, then top with the tomato, onion, and avocado. Finish with a squeeze of lime and a sprinkling of cilantro.

NUTRITION FACTS
FOR 1 SERVING (4 TACOS): **CALORIES:** 352 **PROTEIN:** 10g **CARBS:** 46g **FAT:** 11g

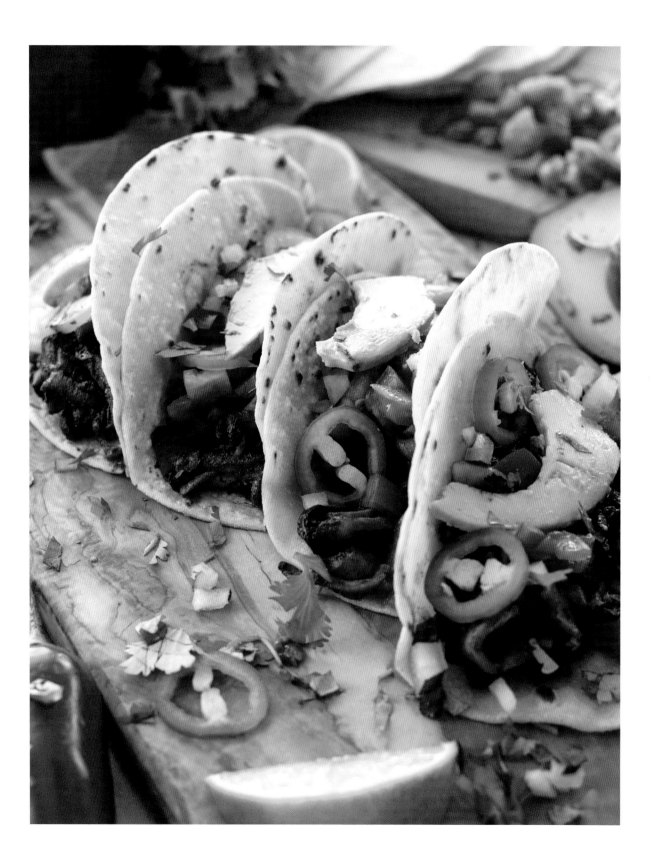

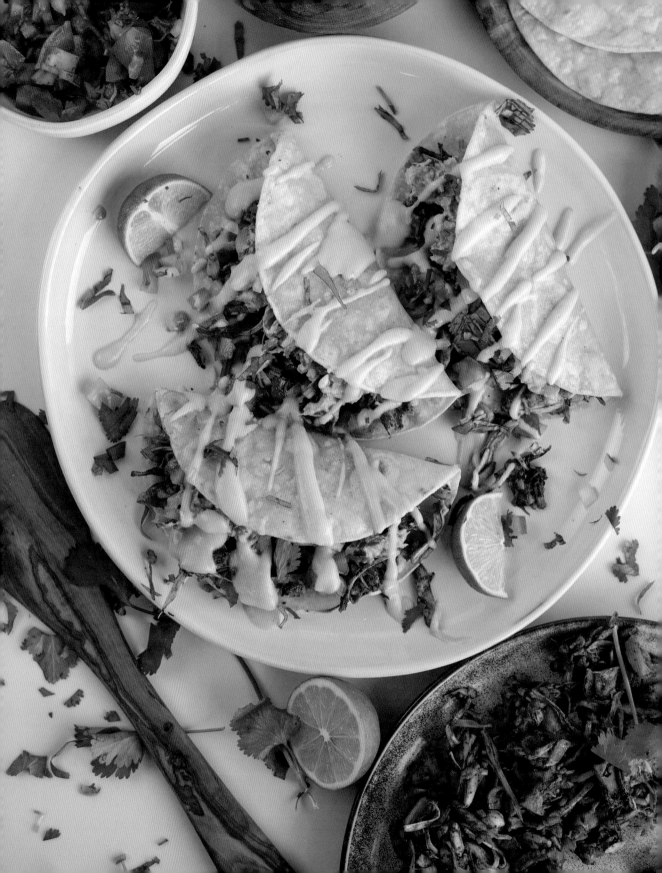

Jackfruit Enchilada Tacos

Saucy, cheesy enchiladas are one of my favorite dishes, but sometimes I want just a few enchiladas, and I don't feel like making an entire casserole of them. This taco version comes together much more quickly but still checks all the enchilada boxes with saucy, meaty jackfruit; Pimento Cheese Sauce; Summer Guac; Pico de Gallo; and Cashew Lime Crema. They're delicious wrapped in a corn tortilla, or if you want even more tacos for fewer calories, use lettuce leaves instead!

Cooking spray (see page 33)

1 (14-ounce) can jackfruit, drained

¼ small yellow onion, diced

Garlic salt, to taste

½ cup fat-free enchilada sauce

5 (6-inch) corn tortillas (60 calories each)

⅓ cup Pimento Cheese Sauce (page 225), warmed

5 tablespoons Summer Guac (page 210)

5 tablespoons Pico de Gallo (page 208)

2 tablespoons Cashew Lime Crema (page 219)

---

1. Heat a large nonstick skillet over medium-high heat. Lightly coat the pan with cooking spray and add the jackfruit and onion. Season with a pinch of the garlic salt and cook, stirring, until the onions brown, about 3 minutes. Add the enchilada sauce and continue cooking and stirring until the mixture deepens in color, another 3 minutes.

2. Divide the jackfruit filling among the tortillas and top with the Pimento Cheese Sauce, Summer Guac, Pico de Gallo, and Cashew Lime Crema.

NOTE: You read that correctly: The serving size for this recipe is 5 (!) tacos. That's because I developed this recipe to get a lot of bang out of your caloric buck. Tacos—or any dish, really—should be enjoyed in abundance, and you can absolutely do that here.

NUTRITION FACTS

FOR 1 SERVING (5 TACOS): CALORIES: 679 PROTEIN: 21g CARBS: 87g FAT: 18g

Loaded Taco Sweet Potato

SERVES
1

Taco fillings aren't usually something you think of putting on a sweet potato, but let me tell you—this sweet and savory combo works. With the natural creaminess of the potato blending with the beans, Summer Guac, and Poblano Cheese Sauce, plus the bright, fresh Cashew Lime Crema and Pico de Gallo bringing all the flavors together, you'll never miss that burrito from your favorite Mexican restaurant again. And just when you thought it couldn't get any better, it's the kind of dish that you can easily prep ahead of time.

---

1 medium sweet potato (280g)

¼ cup (43g) canned black beans, drained and rinsed

¼ cup (41g) fresh or canned corn (drained, if canned)

2 tablespoons Summer Guac (page 210)

¼ cup Poblano Cheese Sauce (page 216), warmed

2 tablespoons Cashew Lime Crema (page 219)

¼ cup Pico de Gallo (page 208)

---

1. Preheat the oven to 425°F. Line a baking sheet with parchment paper and set aside.

2. Pierce the sweet potato all over with a knife. Set it on the prepared baking sheet and bake for 45 to 60 minutes, until a knife slides easily into the center.

3. When the sweet potato is cool enough to handle, slice it in half lengthwise and use a fork to fluff the middle. Top each half with the beans, corn, and Summer Guac, then drizzle with the Poblano Cheese Sauce and Cashew Lime Crema. Top with a dollop of Pico de Gallo and dig in.

NUTRITION FACTS

FOR 1 SERVING: CALORIES: 529   PROTEIN: 16g   CARBS: 74g   FAT: 14g

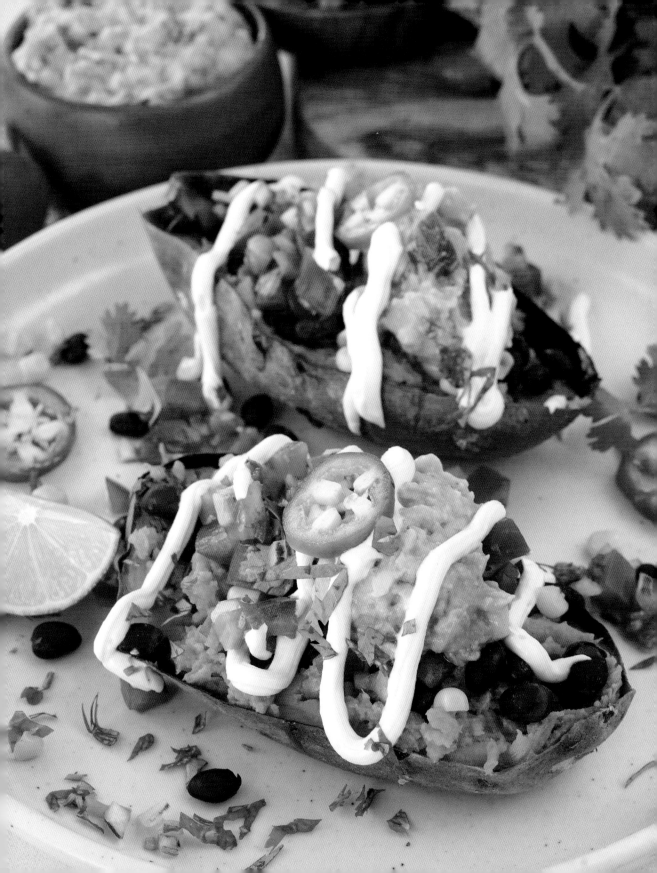

Spinach and Artichoke–Stuffed Mushrooms

SERVES
2
MAKES 5 STUFFED
MUSHROOMS

I took everyone's favorite dip (I think it's safe to say that!) and turned it into a healthy but decadent main that also happens to be beyond easy to whip up. Artichokes and spinach are a classic pairing, and when dolloped onto mashed potatoes, stuffed into roasted mushrooms, and draped in my Garlic Alfredo Sauce, it rivals any non-plant-based version.

---

5 large portobello mushroom
caps (400g), wiped clean

Cooking spray (see page 33, optional)

1 teaspoon garlic salt, divided

½ teaspoon smoked paprika

2 medium russet potatoes (426g),
peeled and cubed

1 cup baby spinach leaves

¼ cup plain, unsweetened almond milk

½ cup canned artichoke hearts in water, drained

1¼ cups Garlic Alfredo Sauce (page 215), warmed

---

1. Preheat the oven to 375°F. Line a baking sheet with parchment paper and set aside.

2. Use your fingers to lightly dampen the mushrooms all over with water, or give them a light coating of cooking spray. (This is just to help the seasonings stick and to keep the mushrooms from drying out in the oven.) Season the mushrooms, top and bottom, with ½ teaspoon of the garlic salt and the smoked paprika and set them face down on the prepared baking sheet. Bake for 15 minutes. Set aside.

3. Meanwhile, put the potatoes in a medium pot and add just enough water to cover. Bring to a boil over medium-high heat, reduce to a simmer, and cook until the potatoes are fork tender, about 15 minutes. Transfer them to a medium bowl and allow them to cool slightly.

4. While the mushrooms and potatoes cook, steam the spinach. Add 2 inches of water to a medium pot with a steamer basket. Bring the water to a simmer over medium heat, add the spinach, cover, and steam until bright green and just tender, about 2 minutes. Transfer to a plate or bowl and set aside.

5. When the potatoes have cooled slightly, use a potato masher or fork to mash them until mostly smooth. Stir in the almond milk and remaining ½ teaspoon of garlic salt until well combined. Fold in the spinach and artichoke hearts and stir until evenly distributed.

6. Top each mushroom with ½ cup of the mashed potato mixture and ¼ cup of the Garlic Alfredo Sauce. Serve warm.

NOTE: For another twist, try this filling stuffed into bell peppers!

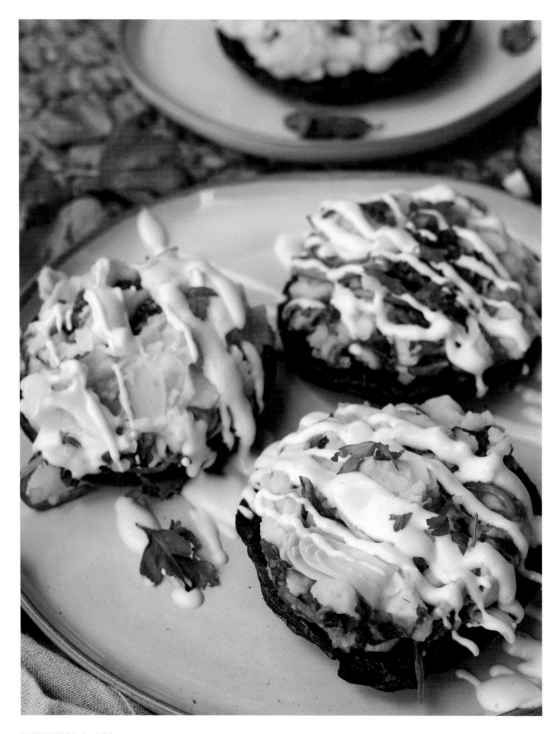

NUTRITION FACTS
FOR 1 SERVING (2½ STUFFED MUSHROOMS) WITH GARLIC ALFREDO SAUCE: CALORIES: 312   PROTEIN: 12g
CARBS: 49g   FAT: 5g

Veggie Supreme Pita Pizzas

SERVES

1

MAKES 2
PIZZAS

I've always said that the best way to eat a low-fat, plant-based diet consistently is to make sure that you always have the option of eating something you truly enjoy. For many people, that includes pizza. That's why I developed this recipe, which uses doughy pita as the crust and calls for heaps of toppings like fresh greens, artichokes, and olives, plus a generous drizzle of decadent Pimento Cheese Sauce. It takes about 10 minutes to pull together, which means you're never more than a moment away from your favorite meal.

2 low-calorie pitas (see page 34)

½ cup marinara sauce (one that's 90 calories or fewer per ½ cup)

1 cup arugula or baby spinach leaves

½ cup canned artichokes in water, drained

¼ cup sliced red onion

1 white mushroom, wiped clean and sliced

1 tablespoon sliced pitted black olives

½ cup Pimento Cheese Sauce (page 225), warmed

1. Preheat the oven to 425°F.

2. Lay the pitas on a baking sheet. Spread ¼ cup of the sauce evenly over each pita and top each with half of the arugula or spinach, artichokes, onion, mushroom, and olives. Bake for 5 minutes, until the vegetables have just softened and the greens are wilted.

3. Drizzle each pizza with half of the Pimento Cheese Sauce and enjoy warm.

NUTRITION FACTS

FOR 1 SERVING (2 PIZZAS):   CALORIES: 360   PROTEIN: 21g   CARBS: 43g   FAT: 9g

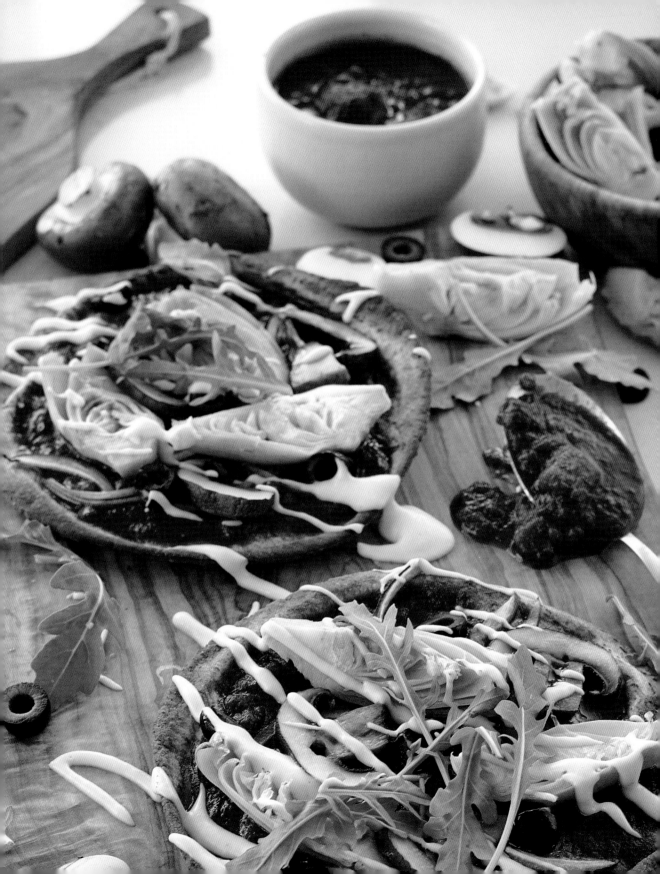

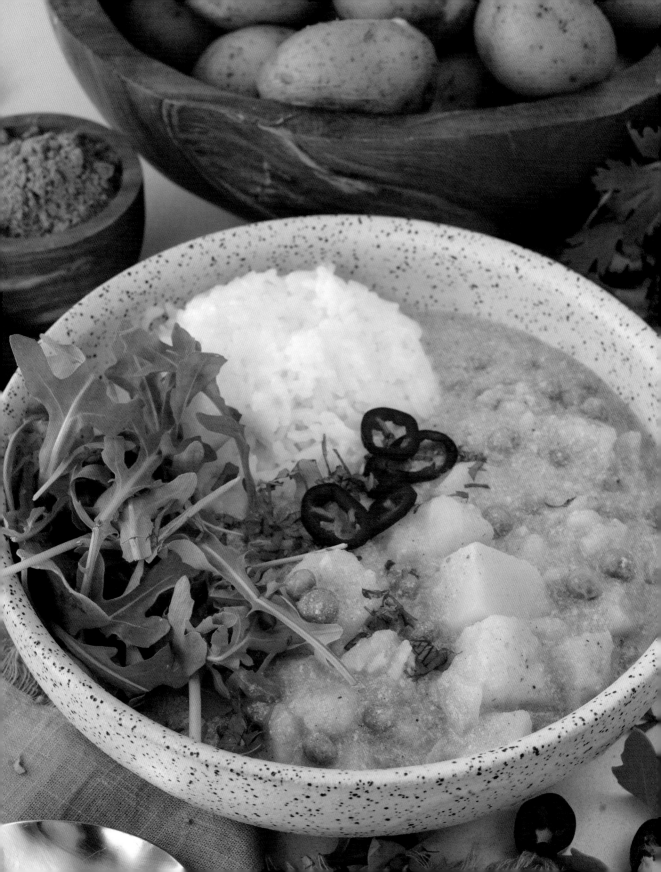

Yellow Potato Curry

I love any dish that's layered with spices, so it tracks that I'm always happy with a curry. And lucky for me, it's easy to take the bold, complex flavors of a curry and add them to an otherwise simple dish. In this case it's potatoes that are scented with the rich, earthy, warming notes of curry powder and garam masala, plus plenty of garlic and ginger. This is a hearty dish that won't leave you feeling weighed down, and it's perfect for busy weekdays and nights because it comes together so quickly.

1. In a medium pot over medium heat, combine the onion, curry powder, garlic, ginger, garam masala, turmeric, and salt. Add the water and cook until the onions are translucent and the spices are fragrant, about 5 minutes. Stir in the almond milk and potatoes and simmer the mixture for 15 minutes, until the potatoes are fork tender.

2. Remove the pot from the heat and stir in the peas, just to defrost them. Adjust the seasoning to taste with a few drops of stevia, a squeeze of lime, and more salt, if needed. Garnish with the cilantro and serve with rice, if desired.

½ cup diced yellow onion

2 teaspoons curry powder

2 teaspoons minced garlic

2 teaspoons minced ginger

1 teaspoon garam masala

¼ teaspoon turmeric powder

¾ teaspoon sea salt, plus more to taste

½ cup water

2 cups plain, unsweetened almond milk

1 large Yukon Gold potato (425g), cubed but not peeled

½ cup frozen peas

Stevia, to taste (I like using coconut-flavored stevia here)

Lime, for serving

1 tablespoon chopped fresh cilantro leaves

1 cup cooked (158g) white or brown rice, for serving (optional)

NOTE: You can enjoy this dish on its own or spoon the curry over white or brown rice.

NUTRITION FACTS

FOR 1 SERVING WITHOUT RICE: **CALORIES:** 516   **PROTEIN:** 15g   **CARBS:** 87g   **FAT:** 6g

FOR 1¾ CUP CURRY WITH 1 CUP (158G) WHITE OR BROWN RICE: **CALORIES:** 463   **PROTEIN:** 11g   **CARBS:** 88g   **FAT:** 4g

Cauliflower Steak Dinner with Mashed Potatoes and Green Beans

SERVES
1
MAKES 3
"STEAKS"

The beauty of cauliflower is that, when roasted, it has a deep, caramelized, savory flavor with a great meaty texture. When I'm feeling nostalgic for steakhouse classics—without the saturated fat and calorie overload—I reach for cauliflower. When sliced into steaks, seasoned with garlic salt, and roasted until crispy, it's absolutely delicious, especially combined with creamy mashed potatoes, garlicky green beans, and a drizzle of vegan Worcestershire sauce.

FOR THE STEAKS
1 medium head of cauliflower
Cooking spray (see page 33)
Garlic salt and freshly ground black pepper, to taste

FOR THE MASHED POTATOES
1 large Yukon gold potato (350g)
¼ cup plain, unsweetened almond milk
½ teaspoon garlic salt, plus more to taste
1 teaspoon chopped chives, for garnish

FOR THE GREEN BEANS
3½ cups fresh or frozen green beans, ends trimmed
⅛ teaspoon garlic salt
Lemon, for serving
1 tablespoon vegan Worcestershire or steak sauce, for serving (optional)

1. Make the steaks: Preheat the oven to 425°F.

2. Slice off the stem at the base of the cauliflower. Sit the cauliflower on the flat end and slice 3 1-inch-thick steaks. You can cook the remaining cauliflower and save it for another meal, or store it raw and make Falafel Cauliflower Pitas (page 120) later in the week.

3. Line a baking sheet with parchment paper. Arrange the slices of cauliflower on the sheet pan and lightly coat each piece on both sides with cooking spray, which will help it brown and not dry out. Season both sides with garlic salt and pepper and roast for 30 minutes, flipping halfway through, until the edges are golden brown and crispy.

4. Meanwhile, make the mashed potatoes: Place the potatoes in a medium pot and add just enough cold water to cover. Bring to a boil over medium-high heat, then reduce to a simmer. Cook until the potatoes are fork tender, about 15 minutes. Transfer the potatoes to a medium bowl and use a potato masher or fork to mash them. Add the almond milk and garlic salt and mix to combine. Adjust the seasoning with more garlic salt (if desired), sprinkle with the chives, and set aside.

NUTRITION FACTS
FOR 1 SERVING: CALORIES: 534   PROTEIN: 24g   CARBS: 88g   FAT: 3g

5. While the potatoes boil, make the green beans: Add 1 inch of water to a medium pot. Put a steamer basket in the pot and bring to a simmer over medium heat. Place the green beans in the steamer basket, cover, and steam until bright green and just tender, 3 to 5 minutes. Transfer the green beans to a medium bowl and toss them with the garlic salt. Finish with a squeeze of lemon.

6. Serve the steaks with the mashed potatoes, green beans, and Worcestershire or steak sauce for dipping, if desired.

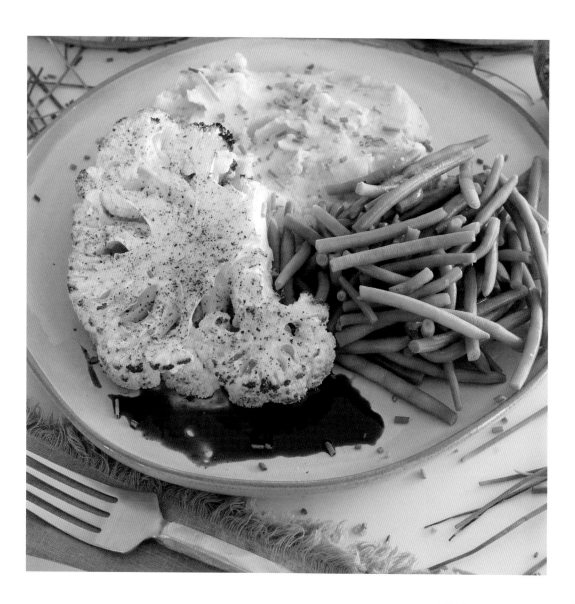

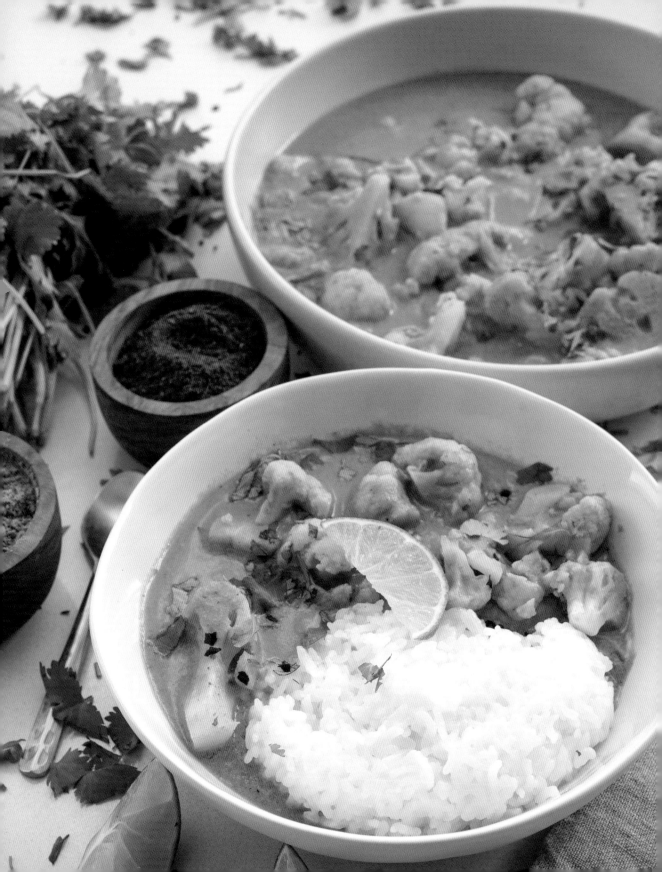

Cauliflower Masala

SERVES
2

If you love Indian food as much as I do, then you've probably had—and been equally obsessed with—chicken tikka masala. You won't be surprised to know that it gets its signature richness from heavy cream and its heartiness from animal protein, which are also major sources of fat and calories. But the amazing flavor in chicken tikka masala comes from a blend of spices and aromatics, which are the secret weapons for making healthy dishes that have complex flavors but that are, in fact, simple to make. By subbing in cauliflower for the chicken and almond milk for the cream, you can easily whip this dish up anytime the craving for something big, bold, and satisfying strikes.

1 (14.5-ounce) can diced tomatoes

½ medium yellow onion

2 teaspoons minced garlic

1 teaspoon minced ginger or
¼ teaspoon dried ginger

1½ teaspoons tikka masala powder

1½ teaspoons curry powder

1 teaspoon sea salt, or more to taste

1 medium head of cauliflower, stemmed
and chopped (about 7 cups or 650g)

2 cups unsweetened almond milk

¼ cup chopped fresh cilantro leaves

Stevia, to taste

Lime, for serving

2 cups (316g) cooked white or brown
rice, for serving (optional)

1. In a blender, combine the tomatoes, onion, garlic, and ginger and blend until smooth. Transfer to a large pot set over medium-high heat. Add the tikka masala powder, curry powder, and salt, and simmer until the sauce thickens slightly, stirring occasionally, about 4 minutes.

2. Add the cauliflower and almond milk and cook until the cauliflower is tender, 10 to 12 minutes. Remove the pot from the heat and stir in the cilantro, stevia, and a squeeze of lime. The dish should have a light, sweet flavor. Adjust the seasoning with more salt, if needed, and serve over rice, if desired.

NUTRITION FACTS
FOR 1 SERVING OF MASALA WITH NO RICE: CALORIES: 203   PROTEIN: 10g   CARBS: 23g   FAT: 4g
FOR 1 SERVING OF MASALA WITH 2 CUPS (316G) WHITE OR BROWN RICE: CALORIES: 614   PROTEIN: 19g
CARBS: 111g   FAT: 5g

Vegan Crab Cakes

SERVES
2
MAKES 7 VEGAN
CRAB CAKES

If you're a seafood lover like I am and are missing those flavors on your plant-based journey, then consider this my gift to you. My stepdad, who isn't interested in a plant-based diet at all, can't get enough of these crispy, creamy cakes, which I think is the best proof of just how good they are. Between the Old Bay seasoning, capers, and my Remoulade sauce, you'd swear you were eating the real thing!

1 (15-ounce) can chickpeas, drained and rinsed

1 (14-ounce) can hearts of palm
packed in water, drained

⅓ cup minced red onion

⅓ cup minced red bell pepper

¼ cup chopped fresh parsley leaves

1 tablespoon Dijon mustard

1 tablespoon brined capers, drained

2½ teaspoons Old Bay seasoning

1 teaspoon fresh lemon juice

1 teaspoon chopped fresh dill

½ teaspoon kelp granules

½ cup panko bread crumbs

Cooking spray (see page 33, optional)

Remoulade (page 222), for serving (optional)

1. In the bowl of a food processor, combine the chickpeas, hearts of palm, onion, bell pepper, parsley, Dijon, capers, Old Bay, lemon juice, dill, and kelp granules. Pulse until the chickpeas are well broken up. Use a spatula to fold in the bread crumbs until evenly distributed.

2. Scoop a loose ½ cup of the filling and use your hands to form it into a ½-inch-thick patty.

3. Heat a large nonstick skillet over medium heat. If you like, you can coat it with cooking spray to encourage even cooking, but it isn't necessary. Add the patties, working in batches if necessary so as not to crowd the pan. Cook until the first side is golden brown, about 3 minutes, then flip and repeat on the other side. Serve with the Remoulade, if desired.

NUTRITION FACTS

FOR 3½ PATTIES WITH NO REMOULADE: CALORIES: 287   PROTEIN: 15g   CARBS: 38g   FAT: 5g

FOR 3½ PATTIES WITH 4 TABLESPOONS REMOULADE: CALORIES: 397   PROTEIN: 18g   CARBS: 46g   FAT: 12g

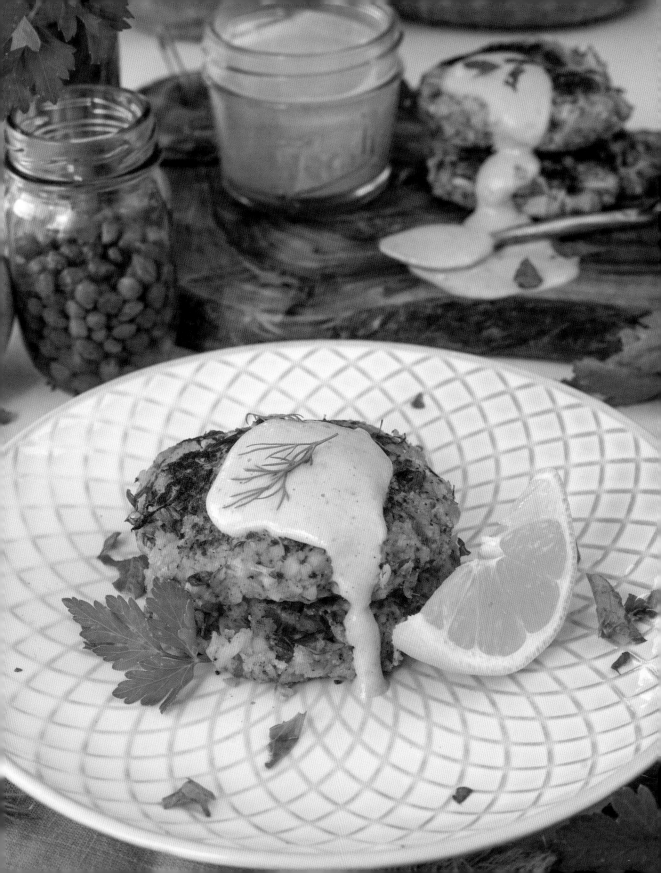

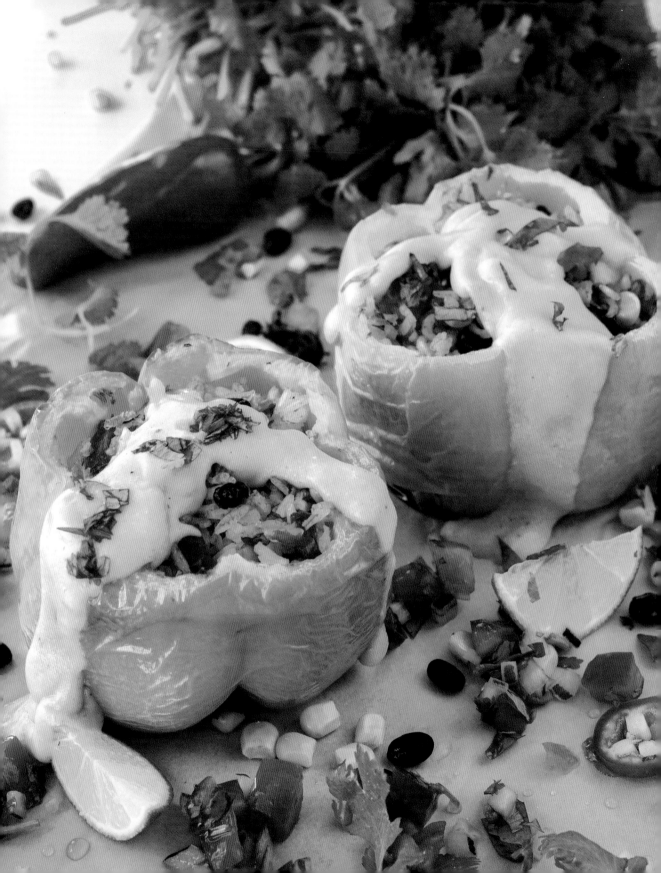

Cilantro-Lime Stuffed Peppers

SERVES
1
MAKES 3 STUFFED
PEPPERS

I don't know if I'm supposed to admit this, but of all the recipes in this book, these stuffed peppers are my favorite. They're fun to put together because the peppers make cute little cups; they're full of protein from the beans and rice; they burst with my favorite Mexican-inspired flavors; and, when smothered in my Poblano Cheese Sauce, they're rich and satisfying. This is also an easy recipe to prep for the week—just throw a batch together, store them in the fridge covered with plastic wrap, and put them right in the oven (uncovered) whenever you're craving them.

---

3 large bell peppers (any color)

1 cup (159g) cooked white or brown rice

¼ cup (43g) canned black beans, drained and rinsed

¼ cup (41g) fresh or canned corn (drained, if canned)

3 tablespoons store-bought or homemade salsa

2 tablespoons chopped fresh cilantro leaves

1 teaspoon fresh lime juice

Garlic salt, to taste

¾ cup Poblano Cheese Sauce (page 216), warmed

---

1. Preheat the oven to 425°F. Line a baking sheet with parchment paper and set aside.

2. Slice off the tops of the bell peppers and use a spoon to scoop out and discard the ribs and seeds. Set the peppers aside.

3. In a medium bowl, mix together the rice, beans, corn, salsa, cilantro, and lime juice. Season to taste with the garlic salt. Divide the filling among the peppers, then arrange them on the prepared baking sheet. Roast for 25 minutes, until the peppers have softened and are beginning to brown.

4. Top the peppers with the Poblano Cheese Sauce and enjoy.

NUTRITION FACTS
FOR 1 SERVING (3 PEPPERS): CALORIES: 563 PROTEIN: 18g CARBS: 93g FAT: 8g

Mexican Hash Brown Bake

SERVES
1

I could list the many reasons why you should make this dish, but I think I'll leave it at this: hash browns plus cheese sauce baked casserole-style. Do I really need to say more? To make it a little more nourishing and a whole lot more filling, I've added a heap of sautéed vegetables, which, when combined with the crunchy hash brown bits and decadent cheese sauce, are enough to appease the biggest of appetites. I think we both know you'll be making this dish on repeat.

---

2 cups (420g) oil-free frozen hash browns (I like Walmart and Kroger brands, as well as Cascadian Farms), thawed

Cooking spray (see page 33, optional)

1 cup (2½ ounces) white mushrooms, diced

1 cup diced zucchini

½ cup yellow onion, diced

½ cup Poblano Cheese Sauce (page 216), plus an additional ¼ cup, warmed

¼ cup chopped fresh cilantro leaves

¼ teaspoon garlic salt, plus more to taste

---

1. Preheat the oven to 425°F.

2. Put the thawed hash browns in a medium bowl and set aside.

3. Heat a large nonstick skillet over medium-high heat. If you like, you can coat it with cooking spray to encourage the vegetables to brown, but it isn't necessary. Add the mushrooms, zucchini, and onion and cook until soft and beginning to brown, 8 to 10 minutes. If the vegetables start to stick, you can add a splash of water.

4. Transfer the vegetables to the bowl with the hash browns. Add ½ cup of the Poblano Cheese Sauce, the cilantro, and the garlic salt and stir to mix well. Taste and add more garlic salt, if desired.

5. Scoop the mixture into a small, oven-safe casserole dish. (I use one that's 6 x 8 inches; anything larger will spread the mixture too thin.) Bake for 20 minutes until warmed through and beginning to brown. Top with the remaining ¼ cup Poblano Cheese Sauce and serve.

NUTRITION FACTS
FOR 1 RECIPE: CALORIES: 551 PROTEIN: 18g CARBS: 96g FAT: 8g

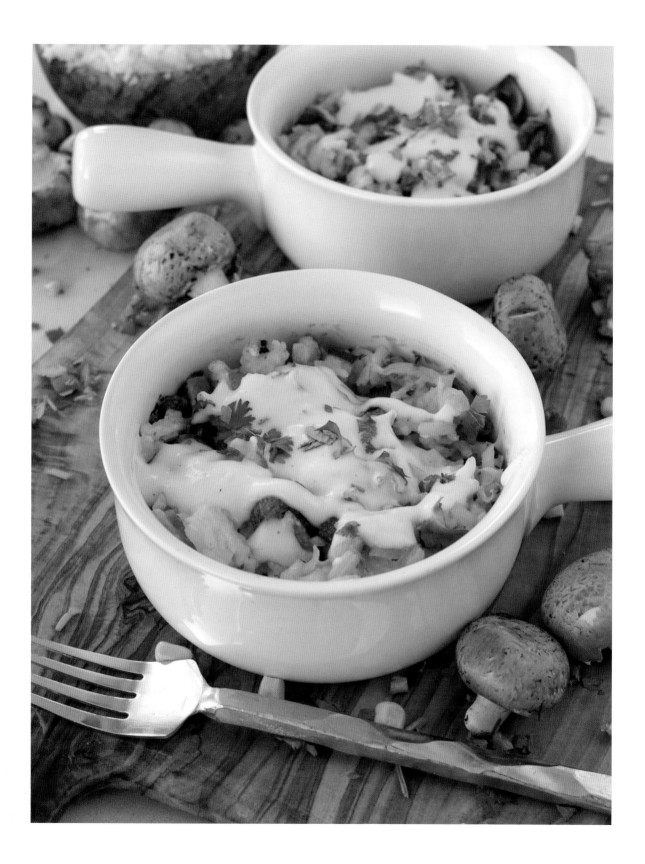

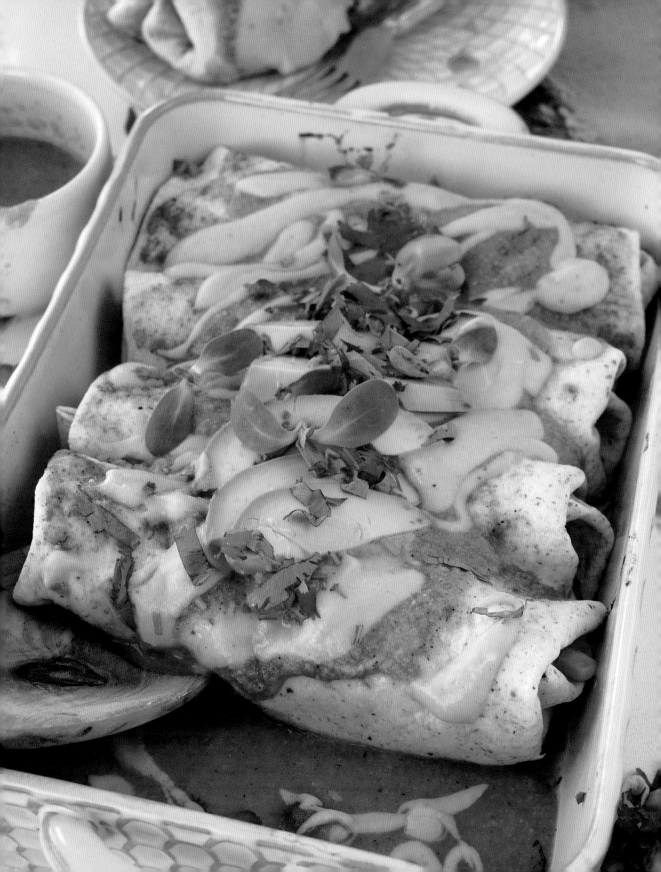

Cheesy Poblano Enchiladas

SERVES
1
MAKES 4
ENCHILADAS

You can create delicious, satisfying enchiladas that are as cheesy and gooey as the best of them—when you start with a base of calorie-dense foods like vegetables and beans, then pack in the flavor with fresh herbs and homemade vegan condiments. You'll be amazed by what a drizzle of store-bought enchilada sauce plus a dollop of my Poblano Cheese Sauce does for this dish!

Cooking spray (see page 33, optional)
1 medium zucchini, diced (about 2 cups)
1 red bell pepper, seeded and diced (1 cup)
¾ cup diced yellow onion
¾ cup low-fat or fat-free green enchilada sauce
½ cup (86g) canned pinto beans, drained and rinsed
**¼ cup (41g) fresh or canned corn
(drained, if canned)**
⅓ cup chopped fresh cilantro leaves
4 (10-inch) flour tortillas (see page 34)
½ cup Poblano Cheese Sauce (page 216)
¼ small avocado (25g), for serving (optional)
**Cashew Lime Crema (page 219),
for serving (optional)**

---

1. Preheat the oven to 375°F.

2. Heat a large nonstick skillet over medium-high heat. If you like, you can coat it with cooking spray to encourage even cooking, but it isn't necessary. Add the zucchini, bell pepper, and onion and sauté until the vegetables are soft and just beginning to brown, 8 to 10 minutes. If the vegetables start to stick, you can add a splash of water.

3. In a medium bowl, combine the sautéed vegetables with ½ cup of the enchilada sauce, the beans, the corn, and the cilantro. Stir to mix well. Lay a tortilla on a work surface and fill it with about one-quarter of the filling. Roll up the tortilla and place it in a 6 x 12-inch baking dish. Continue with the remaining tortillas and filling.

4. Spoon the remaining ¼ cup of enchilada sauce over the enchiladas and bake for 20 minutes, until warmed through. Top the enchiladas with the Poblano Cheese Sauce, plus the avocado and/or Cashew Lime Crema, if desired.

NUTRITION FACTS
FOR 1 SERVING (4 ENCHILADAS), WITHOUT AVOCADO AND CASHEW LIME CREMA: CALORIES: 623   PROTEIN: 27g
CARBS: 88g   FAT: 16g

Pesto Pasta Primavera

SERVES

1

Pesto has a light, herbaceous flavor that makes any dish that much better. However, the traditional method of making it calls for adding Parmesan, nuts, and olive oil—all of which make for a very calorie-dense sauce. Luckily, no one said you're required to add those ingredients in order to get a bright sauce. My version is low in fat and calories but still creamy and fresh. Drizzle it over a simple bowl of whole-grain pasta and zucchini, and dinner (or lunch) is done.

---

3 ounces uncooked whole-grain pasta

Cooking spray (see page 33)

2 cups zucchini sliced into half-moons (from 1 large zucchini)

Garlic salt, to taste

⅔ cup Pesto Dressing (page 196)

3 teaspoons (9g) plant-based Parmesan cheese (see page 172), for serving (optional; adds 24 calories)

---

1. Fill a medium pot with water and bring to a boil over medium-high heat. Add the pasta and cook according to the package instructions. Drain and set aside.

2. While the pasta cooks, heat a large nonstick skillet over medium-high heat. If you like, you can coat it with cooking spray to encourage the zucchini to brown, but it isn't necessary. Add the zucchini and season with a pinch of garlic salt. Cook, stirring occasionally, until the zucchini begins to brown, about 3 minutes. If it starts to stick, you can add a splash of water. Remove the pan from the heat.

3. In a medium bowl, combine the pasta with the zucchini. Top with the Pesto Dressing and toss to coat. Sprinkle with the Parmesan, if desired, and serve.

NUTRITION FACTS

FOR 1 SERVING WITHOUT PARMESAN: CALORIES: 470 PROTEIN: 20g CARBS: 67g FAT: 12g

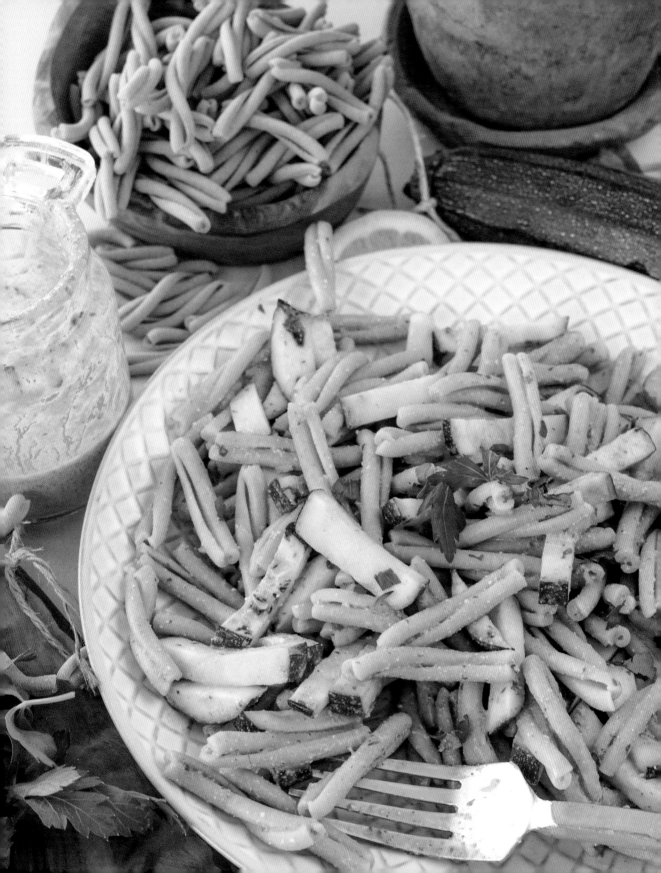

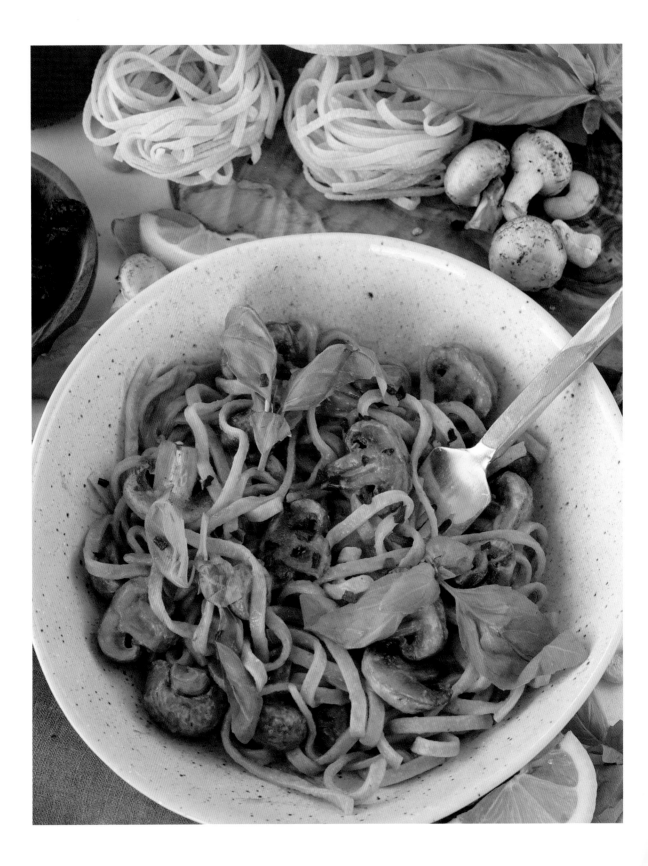

Creamy Roasted Pepper Pasta

SERVES
1

One of the most mind-blowing discoveries I made when transitioning to a high-carbohydrate, low-fat diet was that I could eat pasta and lose weight. I still sometimes have to pinch myself! While I'd be happy most days with a big, steaming bowl of plain pasta, that can get a little old. So, I came up with this dish, which combines a creamy roasted red pepper sauce with meaty mushrooms and fresh basil. It truly is pasta at its finest.

---

4 ounces uncooked whole-grain pasta
Cooking spray (see page 33, optional)
8 ounces baby bella mushrooms,
wiped clean and quartered
½ cup Roasted Red Pepper Sauce (page 213)
1 tablespoon chopped fresh basil leaves

---

1. Cook the pasta according to package instructions, drain, and put in a medium bowl. Set aside.

2. Heat a large nonstick skillet over medium-high heat. If you like, you can coat it with cooking spray to encourage the mushrooms to brown, but it isn't necessary. Add the mushrooms and cook until soft and beginning to brown, about 8 minutes. If they start to stick, you can add a splash of water.

3. Transfer the mushrooms to the bowl with the pasta. Drizzle the Roasted Red Pepper Sauce over the top and toss to coat well. Top with the chopped basil and serve.

NUTRITION FACTS
FOR 1 SERVING: **CALORIES:** 540 **PROTEIN:** 25g **CARBS:** 89g **FAT:** 7g

Spring Alfredo Pasta

SERVES
1

I think we can all agree that pasta is the ultimate comfort food, but what always surprises people is when I tell them that it can be healthy, too! The trick is to use a whole-grain pasta so you're getting high-quality carbohydrate energy, while also working in lots of veggies for an extra punch of nutrients and fiber. When it comes to the sauce, it's all about the right swaps and seasonings, which is what makes my Garlic Alfredo Sauce so easy to love.

---

3 ounces uncooked whole-grain pasta

1 small zucchini (130g), thinly sliced, or 1 cup zoodles

2 asparagus spears, tough ends trimmed and cut into 1-inch pieces

1 cup packed fresh baby spinach or arugula

½ cup Garlic Alfredo Sauce (page 215), warmed

⅛ teaspoon garlic salt, plus more to taste

Freshly ground black pepper, to taste

---

1. Fill a medium pot with water and bring to a boil over medium-high heat. Cook the pasta according to package instructions. Drain and set aside.

2. While the pasta cooks, bring 2 inches of water to a simmer in another medium pot with a fitted lid. Place a steamer basket in the pot and add the zucchini and asparagus. Cover and steam for 3 to 5 minutes, until the vegetables are bright green and tender but not mushy. Alternatively, you could add them to a microwave-safe container with 1 tablespoon of water, cover, and microwave for 3 minutes.

3. In a large bowl, add the pasta, zucchini, and spinach or arugula and gently toss to combine. (The heat from the pasta and zucchini will wilt the spinach.) Pour the Garlic Alfredo Sauce over the top and gently toss again to coat. Season with the garlic salt and a few twists of pepper, adding more garlic salt if desired.

NUTRITION FACTS

FOR 1 SERVING: **CALORIES:** 404   **PROTEIN:** 16g   **CARBS:** 67g   **FAT:** 6g

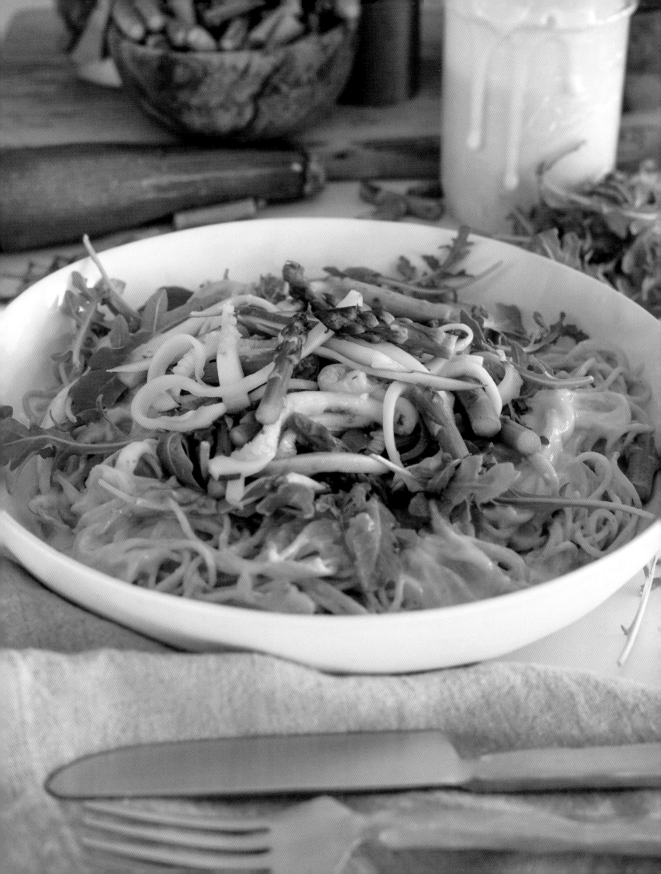

Lean Lasagna

SERVES
2

"Lasagna" and "lean" aren't usually found together in a sentence. It was my goal, however, to deliver a recipe that would feel as hearty and soothing as the OG comfort-food dish and yet still be low in calories and fat. I discovered that a mix of tofu and nutritional yeast is a dead ringer for ricotta cheese, and when blended with sautéed mushrooms and artichokes, it gives you a flavorful baked dish that nourishes you, body and soul.

Cooking spray (see page 33, optional)

16 ounces white mushrooms, wiped clean and chopped

⅔ block (370g/100 oz) extra-firm tofu

2 cups packed fresh baby spinach leaves

1 cup (170g) canned artichoke hearts, drained and chopped

¼ cup nutritional yeast

2 tablespoons fresh lemon juice

1 teaspoon garlic salt, plus more to taste

1 teaspoon Italian seasoning

¼ teaspoon onion powder

¼ teaspoon garlic powder

3 cups fat-free marinara sauce (see page 33)

8 to 12 sheets no-bake lasagna noodles (288g; use gluten-free, if desired)

Grated vegan Parmesan, optional (see page 172)

---

1. Preheat the oven to 375°F.

2. Heat a large nonstick skillet over medium-high heat. If you like, you can coat it with cooking spray to encourage even cooking, but it isn't necessary. Add the mushrooms and sauté until soft, about 6 minutes. If they start to stick, you can add a splash of water.

3. In a food processor, combine the sautéed mushrooms with the tofu, spinach, artichoke hearts, nutritional yeast, lemon juice, garlic salt, Italian seasoning, onion powder, and garlic powder. Pulse a few times until the mixture achieves a smooth, ricotta-like consistency. Adjust the seasonings with more garlic salt, if desired.

4. Spread a spoonful of the marinara over the bottom of an 8 x 12-inch casserole dish. Lay down the first noodle, followed by a layer of ½ cup of the tofu mixture. Add a spoonful of the mari-

NUTRITION FACTS
FOR 1 SERVING WITHOUT PARMESAN: **CALORIES:** 627 **PROTEIN:** 47g **CARBS:** 75g **FAT:** 10g

nara, and then another noodle layer. Repeat the layers until you've run out of noodles, reserving ½ cup of the marinara. Pour ¼ cup water around the edges of the dish so it runs to the bottom of the casserole, cover the dish with foil, and bake for 45 to 55 minutes, until the noodles are cooked through.

5. Allow the lasagna to cool slightly before topping with the remaining ½ cup of marinara and sprinkling with vegan Parmesan, if desired. Slice and serve.

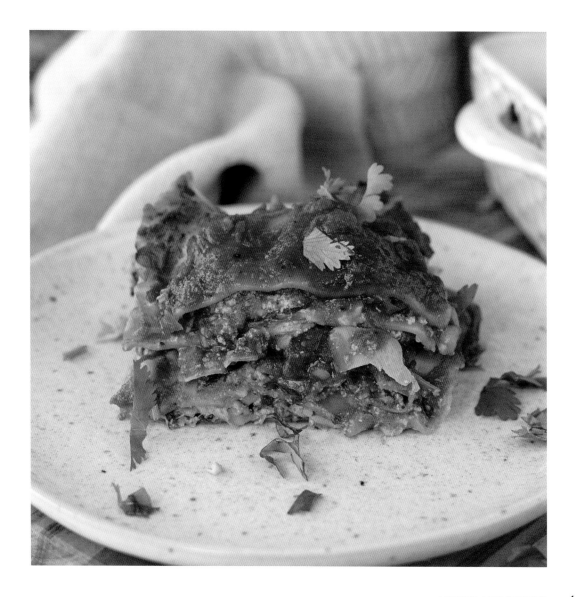

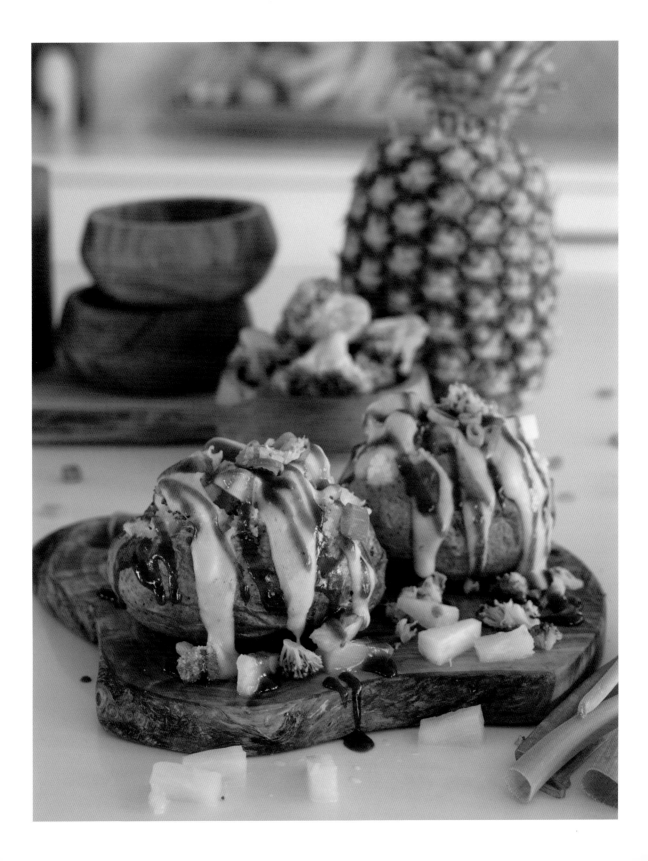

Hawaiian Potatoes

SERVES
1

Potatoes are the ultimate blank canvas—their mild (always-comforting) flavor pairs with just about anything, and they're so satisfying to eat that whatever sauce or veggie medley you decide to top them with instantly becomes a meal. When I thought about my favorite flavor combinations to add to this dish, my mind immediately went to the sweet, tangy pairing of pineapple and barbecue sauce . . . followed by a decadent dollop of my Pimento Cheese Sauce. I added some broccoli for good measure—because balance—but the overall aesthetic of this dish is all indulgent, all the time.

---

2 medium russet potatoes (500g)

2 cups (155g) fresh or frozen broccoli florets

½ cup (47g) canned or fresh pineapple tidbits (see Note)

1 scallion, sliced (white and green parts)

½ cup Pimento Cheese Sauce (page 225), warmed

1 to 2 tablespoons of your favorite barbecue sauce

NOTE: If using canned pineapple—which I'm a big fan of, for saving time—be sure to look for a brand that cans it in juice and not syrup.

1. Boil or bake your potatoes. If baking, preheat the oven to 425°F. Pierce the potatoes all over and bake on a baking sheet for 45 minutes, until fork tender. If boiling, add the potatoes to a medium or large pot. Add just enough water to cover, cover with the lid, and bring to a boil over medium-high heat. Boil for 20 to 25 minutes, until fork tender. If using an Instant Pot, insert the steaming basket and add the potatoes. Add just enough water to cover and close with the lid. Use the Steam function to cook for 18 minutes. Release the pressure manually.

2. While the potatoes cook, bring 2 inches of water to a simmer in a medium pot with a fitted lid. Place a steamer basket in the pot and add the broccoli. Cover the pot and steam for 6 minutes, until the broccoli is bright green and tender but not mushy. Alternatively, you could add the broccoli to a microwave-safe container with 1 tablespoon of water, cover, and microwave for 4 minutes.

3. Slice the potatoes open as you would a baked potato, or mash them. Top with the steamed broccoli, pineapple, scallion, Pimento Cheese Sauce, and barbecue sauce.

NUTRITION FACTS

FOR 1 SERVING: CALORIES: 634   PROTEIN: 16g   CARBS: 121g   FAT: 4g

Mushroom Stroganoff

SERVES
2

When I was a kid, beef stroganoff was one of my favorite recipes that my mom would make for us. It was the perfect rich, creamy dish to savor at the end of a long day at school. When I got older, I found out it was also one of my mom's favorite recipes to cook because it was an easy way to fill bellies without a lot of effort. Plus, it's always a major bonus when everyone at the table is happy, kids and adults. I've played around with the recipe to make it plant-based, but I assure you that this is every bit as soothing and satisfying as the original.

6 ounces uncooked pasta of your choice

½ cup plain, unsweetened almond milk

¼ cup raw cashews (130g)

Cooking spray (see page 33, optional)

8 ounces baby bella mushrooms, sliced or quartered

½ small yellow onion (110g), diced

2 tablespoons vegan Worcestershire sauce

Garlic salt, to taste

Ground black pepper, to taste

1 tablespoon chopped fresh parsley leaves, for garnish

Grated plant-based Parmesan, for serving (optional; see Note)

1. Fill a medium pot with water and bring to a boil over medium-high heat. Add the pasta and cook according to package instructions. Drain and set aside.

2. While the pasta cooks, start the sauce. In a blender, combine the almond milk and cashews and blend until smooth. Set aside.

3. Heat a large nonstick skillet over medium-high heat. If you like, you can coat it with cooking spray to encourage even cooking, but it isn't necessary. Add the mushrooms and onion and sauté until they have softened and are beginning to brown, 8 to 10 minutes. If they start to stick, you can add a splash of water. Remove the pan from the heat and stir in the cashew mixture and the Worcestershire sauce.

4. Add the pasta and toss until well coated. Season with garlic salt and pepper to taste, then garnish with the parsley. Serve with a sprinkling of the Parmesan, if desired.

> NOTE: This dish is extremely delicious on its own, but adding a sprinkling of plant-based Parmesan (I like Violife) at the end makes it even more decadent. (Just be sure to add an extra 24 calories for 9g of cheese.)

NUTRITION FACTS

FOR 1 SERVING, NOT INCLUDING PARMESAN: CALORIES: 450 PROTEIN: 19g CARBS: 67g FAT: 11g

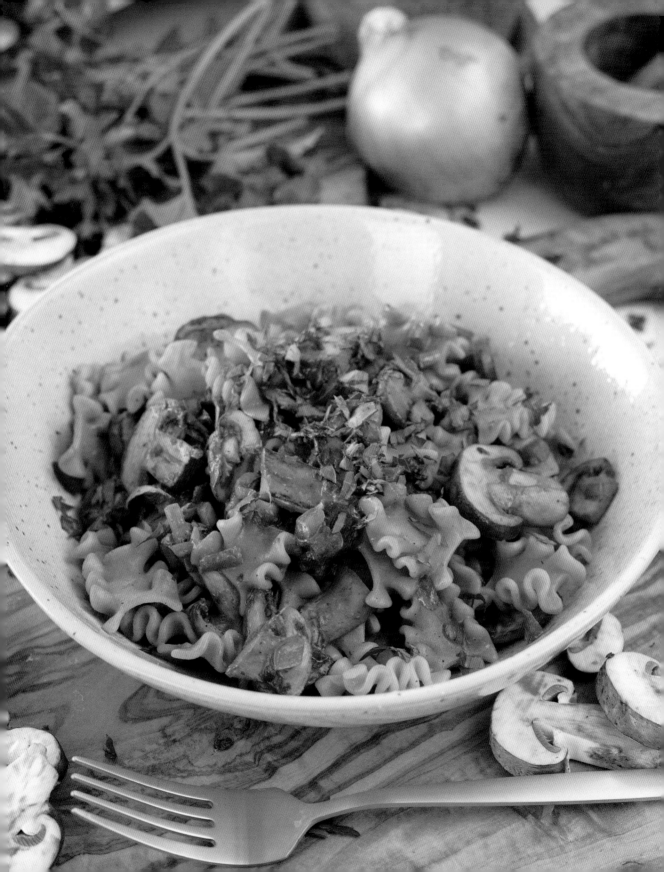

Smoky Sweet Chili

SERVES
1

A warm bowl of good chili is always undeniably comforting. And it doesn't need ground beef or cheese to make it special or satisfying. To me, a quality chili is one with tons of smoky-sweet flavor from a blend of spices, plus hearty texture from beans and tomatoes. Of course, it never hurts to top it off with something cool and creamy, which is why I've included a drizzle of my Cashew Lime Crema. This may look like a lot of ingredients at first glance, but I bet you already have many of them in your pantry, and you're pretty much just tossing 'em all in the pot!

1 (15-ounce) can chili beans, drained
1 (14-ounce) can diced tomatoes
½ small yellow onion (110g), diced
1 tablespoon minced garlic
1 tablespoon ketchup
1 tablespoon maple syrup
1 to 2 teaspoons chipotle powder (depending on how much spice you like; optional)
1 teaspoon smoked paprika
½ teaspoon chili powder
¼ teaspoon garlic salt, plus more to taste
Lime, for serving
Chopped fresh cilantro, for serving
3 tablespoons Cashew Lime Crema (page 219)

In a medium pot over medium-high heat, combine the beans, tomatoes, onion, garlic, ketchup, maple syrup, chipotle powder (if using), paprika, chili powder, and garlic salt. Bring the mixture to a boil, reduce to a simmer, and cook for 5 to 10 minutes, until heated through. Season with more garlic salt, if needed. Serve with a squeeze of lime, a sprinkle of cilantro, and a drizzle of Cashew Lime Crema.

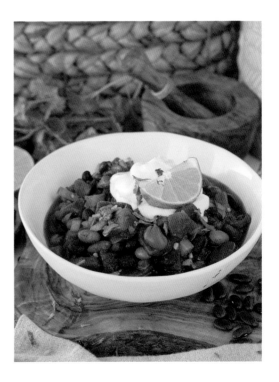

NUTRITION FACTS
FOR 1 SERVING: CALORIES: 657   PROTEIN: 26g   CARBS: 88g   FAT: 13g

Curry Potato and Apple Bowl

SERVES
1

My mom isn't the only one in the family who's famous for her chicken salad (see page 128)—my sweet mother-in-law also has a fan favorite. Her secret is adding grapes, apples, and curry powder, which give the salad an irresistible sweet and spicy flavor and great texture. The apples are crisp and juicy and add a pop of sweetness. For my plant-based twist, I swap creamy cooked potatoes for the chicken and yogurt for the mayo, but the effect is still deliciously the same.

3 medium Yukon Gold potatoes (440g)

½ cup plain, unsweetened plant-based yogurt

1 tablespoon fresh lemon juice

1 tablespoon chopped fresh cilantro

¾ teaspoon curry powder

¼ teaspoon garlic salt, plus more to taste

2 drops of stevia, plus more to taste

Freshly ground black pepper, to taste

4 cups spring greens or other lettuces, such as Bibb or butter

½ cup fuji apple, cored and diced

½ cup red grapes or other seedless grapes, sliced

⅓ cup finely diced celery

¼ cup finely diced red onion

1 tablespoon (9g) chopped walnuts

NOTE: I love this salad over a bed of greens, but you could also use it in a low-calorie wrap (see page 33).

1. Place the potatoes in a small pot and add just enough water to cover. Over medium-high heat, bring the water to a boil, then reduce to a simmer. Cook until the potatoes are fork tender, about 20 minutes. Drain and set aside to cool slightly while you make the rest of the salad.

2. In a small bowl, stir together the yogurt, lemon juice, cilantro, curry powder, and garlic salt. Add 2 drops of stevia and adjust the seasonings with more garlic salt, a few twists of black pepper, or another drop of stevia, if desired.

3. Add the greens to a large bowl and top with the potatoes, apple, grapes, celery, and onion.

4. Drizzle the yogurt mixture over the salad and toss to mix well. Sprinkle with the walnuts and serve.

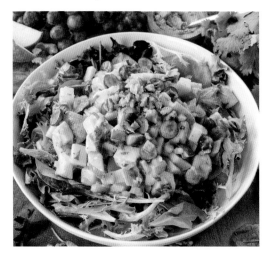

NUTRITION FACTS

FOR 1 SERVING: CALORIES: 592   PROTEIN: 15g   CARBS: 101g   FAT: 11g

Peanut Soba Noodles

SERVES
1

Soba noodles, which are used frequently in Japanese cooking and are made from buckwheat, lend a unique earthy, slightly nutty flavor and satisfying toothsomeness to a dish—in addition to really hitting the spot whenever you're in the mood for a steaming-hot bowlful of noodles. They're especially delicious when tossed with a blend of vegetables—most of which are raw and can therefore be prepped in advance and thrown together in no time—and coated in a creamy, savory peanut sauce. If this is a dish you anticipate wanting to eat multiple times in a week, I highly recommend making a scaled-up batch of the sauce, which will keep for up to 3 days.

FOR THE NOODLES
1 bundle (76g) uncooked soba noodles (see Note)

Cooking spray (see page 33, optional)

1 cup shiitake mushrooms, wiped
clean, stemmed, and sliced

2 tablespoons minced yellow onion

½ cup shredded red cabbage

¼ cup sliced bell pepper

¼ cup shredded carrot

1 scallion, sliced (white and green parts)

2 tablespoons chopped fresh cilantro leaves

Lime, for serving

FOR THE PEANUT SAUCE
4 tablespoons powdered peanut butter

2 tablespoon fresh lime juice

1 tablespoon maple syrup

2 teaspoons low-sodium soy sauce

2 teaspoons minced garlic

2 teaspoons oil-free chili paste (I like sambal oelek)

¼ teaspoon toasted sesame oil

Pinch of minced fresh or ground ginger

1. Make the noodles: Fill a medium pot with water and bring to a boil over medium-high heat. Add the noodles and cook according to package instructions. Drain, rinse with cold water, and set aside.

2. While the noodles cook, heat a large nonstick skillet over medium-high heat. If you like, you can coat it with cooking spray to encourage even cooking, but it isn't necessary. Add the mushrooms and onion and sauté until the vegetables have softened, 5 minutes. If the vegetables begin to stick, you can add a splash of water. Remove the pan from the heat.

3. Make the sauce: In a medium bowl, stir together the powdered peanut butter, lime juice, maple syrup, soy sauce, garlic, chili paste, toasted sesame oil, and ginger. Add 1 tablespoon of water and stir again to combine.

4. In a large bowl, combine the noodles with the mushrooms and onions, cabbage, pepper, carrot, and scallion. Drizzle the peanut sauce over the top and toss to coat. Finish with a sprinkle of cilantro and a squeeze of lime.

NOTE: You could also use gluten-free noodles for this dish (check the package to ensure that they're made from 100 percent buckwheat) or any pasta that you already have in your pantry.

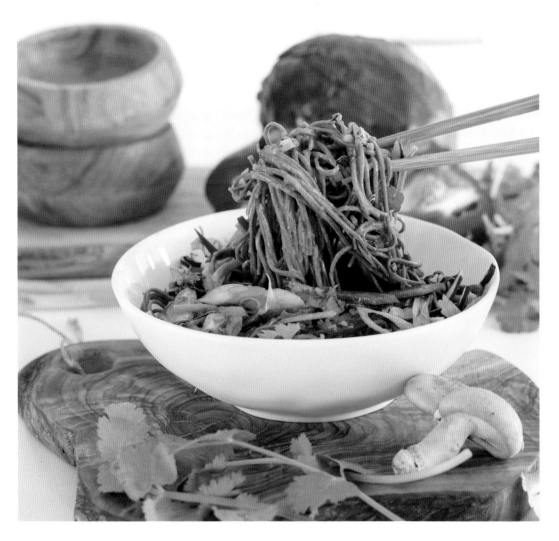

NUTRITION FACTS
FOR 1 SERVING: **CALORIES:** 513   **PROTEIN:** 26g   **CARBS:** 91g   **FAT:** 5g

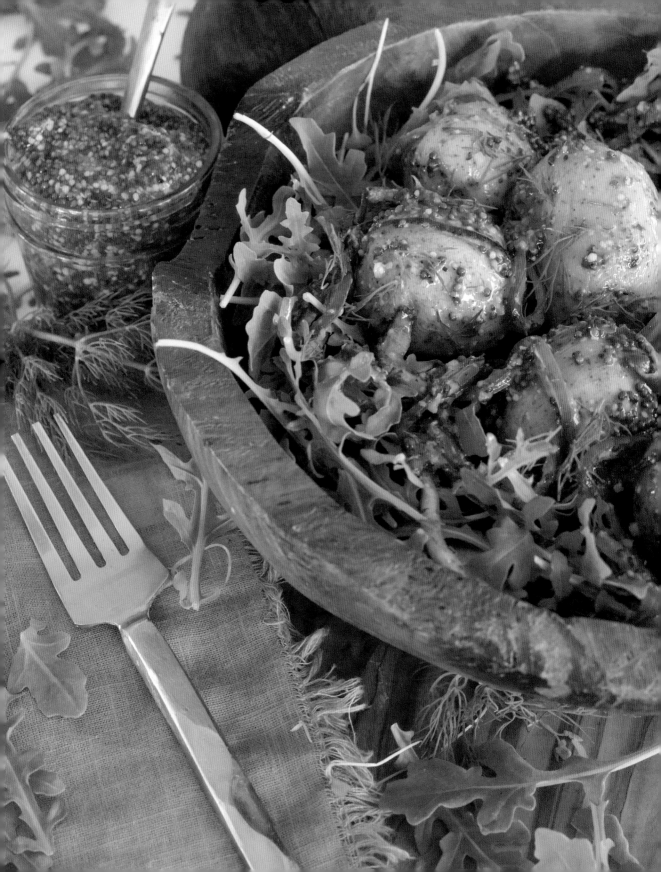

French Potato Salad Bowl

Potato salad often brings to mind the gloppy, mayonnaise-y picnic staple. But in Southern France, potato salad is a whole other story—fresh and light, with tons of herbs and ground mustard. In my version, I also add a little maple syrup for a hint of sweetness to round out the flavors, and it makes for the most perfect meal when scooped over a bed of greens.

---

2 cups baby potatoes (370g)
1 tablespoon coarse-ground mustard
1 tablespoon maple syrup
1 tablespoon fresh lemon juice
½ teaspoon minced garlic
1 tablespoon chopped fresh dill
3 cups arugula or spring greens
½ cup sliced red onion

---

1. Place the potatoes in a small pot and add just enough water to cover. Over medium-high heat, bring the water to a boil, then reduce to a simmer. Cook until the potatoes are fork tender, about 20 minutes. Drain and set aside to cool slightly while you make the rest of the salad.

2. In a small bowl, stir together the mustard, maple syrup, lemon juice, garlic, and dill.

3. Add the greens to a large bowl. Scatter the potatoes over the top, followed by the onion. Drizzle with the dressing and toss well to combine.

NUTRITION FACTS
FOR 1 SERVING: CALORIES: 405   PROTEIN: 9g   CARBS: 80g   FAT: 1g

Teriyaki Bowl

SERVES
1

When people want to know the secret to maintaining a whole-food, plant-based diet, I tell them about the trick that saves me meal after meal: the bowl. They're easy and quick to throw together, are full of filling ingredients, and are meant for layering all your favorite flavors and textures to enjoy together in one bite. This version is always in my rotation because I love the combination of tangy teriyaki sauce with meaty mushrooms—plus I can batch prep almost all the components in advance.

2 cups fresh or frozen broccoli florets
Cooking spray (see page 33 optional)
8 ounces portobello mushroom caps, wiped clean and sliced
Pinch of garlic salt
2 cups (316g) white or brown rice, steamed
4 tablespoons Teriyaki Sauce (page 212)
¼ teaspoon black sesame seeds

1. In a medium pot with a fitted lid, bring 2 inches of water to a simmer. Place the broccoli in a steamer basket and put the basket in the pot. Cover the pot and steam for 5 minutes, until the broccoli is bright green and just tender but not mushy. Alternatively, you can add the broccoli to a microwave-safe container with 1 tablespoon of water, cover, and microwave for 4 minutes. Set aside.

2. Heat a large nonstick skillet over medium heat. If you like, spray the pan with cooking spray, which can encourage the mushrooms to brown but isn't necessary. Add the mushrooms and season them with the garlic salt. Cook until the mushrooms are tender, 5 to 8 minutes. If the mushrooms start to stick, you can add a splash of water. Remove the pan from the heat.

3. In a serving bowl, create a bed of the rice and top with the mushrooms and broccoli. Drizzle with the Teriyaki Sauce and sprinkle with the sesame seeds.

NUTRITION FACTS
FOR 1 SERVING: **CALORIES:** 548 **PROTEIN:** 17g **CARBS:** 109g **FAT:** 3g

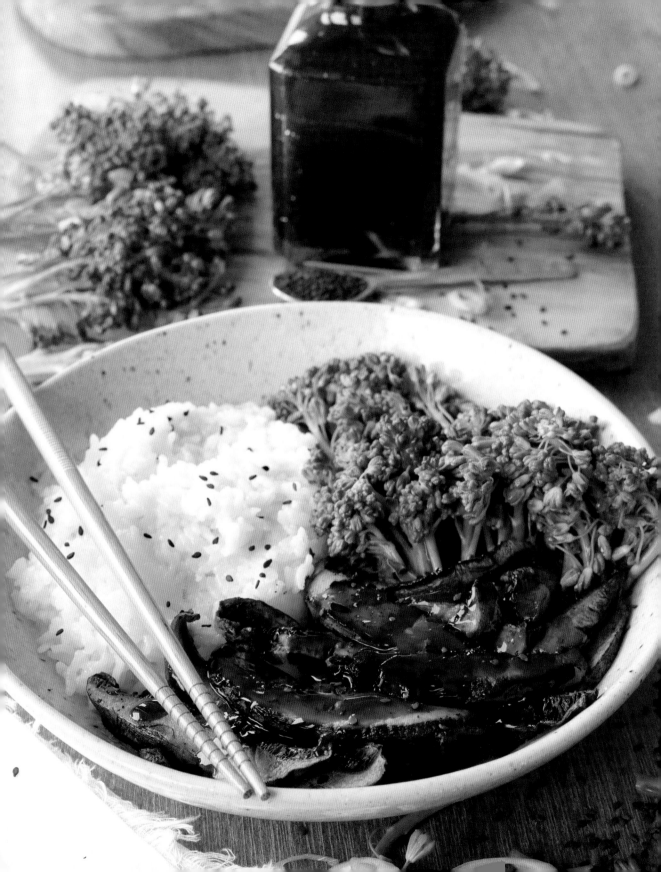

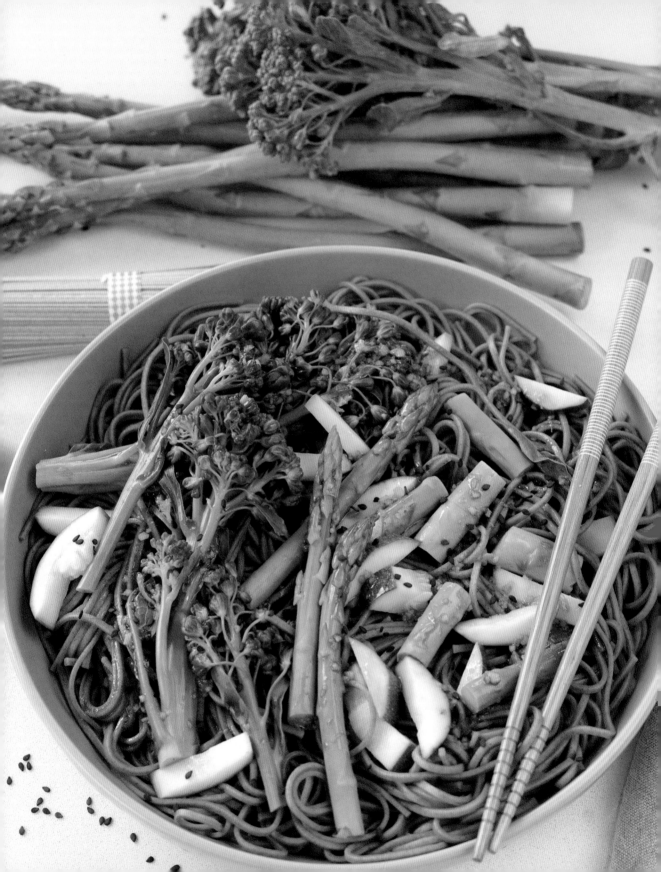

Sesame Ginger Cold Noodle Bowl

SERVES
1

This light, Asian-inspired chilled noodle salad is a refreshing alternative to other low-fuss options such as salads or sandwiches, and you can also whip it up in under 20 minutes. In the time it takes you to quickly cook the noodles and steam the broccolini, you can pull together a delicious dressing that gets deep, savory flavor from toasted sesame oil plus a punch from ginger paste. This recipe scales up nicely and would be great prepped ahead and stored in the fridge for up to 3 days.

1 bundle of soba noodles (78g)

1 small zucchini sliced into half-moons or matchsticks

5 asparagus spears (about ½ bundle), ends trimmed and chopped into bite-size pieces

1 cup broccolini

2 tablespoons low-sodium soy sauce

2 tablespoons seasoned rice vinegar

1 teaspoon ginger paste

1 teaspoon maple syrup

½ teaspoon toasted sesame oil

½ teaspoon minced garlic

Chili flakes, optional

1. Fill a medium pot with water and bring to a boil over medium-high heat. Add the noodles and cook until tender, about 5 minutes. Transfer to a colander, rinse with cold water, and set aside.

2. Meanwhile, add two inches of water to another medium pot and add a basket steamer. Bring to a simmer over medium heat and add the zucchini, asparagus, and broccolini. Cover and steam until all the vegetables are bright green and tender, about 3 minutes. Remove from the heat and set aside.

3. In a small bowl, whisk together the soy sauce, rice vinegar, ginger paste, maple syrup, toasted sesame oil, and garlic until well combined.

4. In a serving bowl, combine the soba noodles and the vegetables. Drizzle with the dressing and toss to coat. Sprinkle with the chili flakes, if desired, and serve.

NUTRITION FACTS
CALORIES: 397   **PROTEIN:** 18g   **CARBS:** 77g   **FAT:** 4g

Fajita Bowl

Don't let this simple recipe fool you; at its core is a viral TikTok sensation. When I posted a video about it, hundreds of thousands of people just about lost their minds over seeing how a meal so low in calories could be so delicious and filling. Between the roasted vegetables seasoned with smoky flavor, the creamy avocado, and the tangy ranch dressing, you're most likely going to join the fan club for this one, too.

---

1 medium Yukon gold potato (325g)
1 red bell pepper, seeded and sliced
1 small red onion (150g), sliced
1 portobello mushroom cap (110g), sliced
½ teaspoon chili powder or fajita/taco seasoning
Smoked paprika, to taste
Garlic salt, to taste
4 cups (80g) spring greens
¼ medium avocado (25g), optional
½ cup Smokehouse Ranch (page 197)
¼ cup chopped fresh cilantro, for garnish, optional
2 teaspoons of your favorite hot sauce, optional

---

1. Place the potato in a small pot and add just enough water to cover. Over medium-high heat, bring the water to a boil, then reduce to a simmer. Cook until the potato is fork tender, about 20 minutes. Drain and set aside to cool slightly.

When cool enough to handle, dice the potato into 1-inch pieces.

2. Preheat the oven to 375°F.

3. Line a baking sheet with parchment paper and add the diced potato, bell pepper, onion, and mushroom. Season with the chili powder and a pinch of smoked paprika and garlic salt. Toss to coat and spread the vegetables evenly over the sheet. Roast for 15 to 20 minutes, until the vegetables are tender and beginning to brown.

4. Add the greens to a large bowl and top with the roasted vegetables. Set the avocado (if using) over the top, followed by the Smokehouse Ranch, cilantro, and hot sauce, if desired.

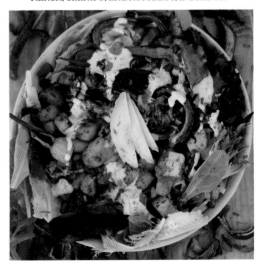

NUTRITION FACTS
FOR 1 SERVING WITH NO AVOCADO: CALORIES: 562 **PROTEIN:** 18g **CARBS:** 75g **FAT:** 19g
FOR 1 SERVING WITH AVOCADO: CALORIES: 604 **PROTEIN:** 18.5g **CARBS:** 75.4g **FAT:** 23g

Chickpea Avocado Bowl

SERVES
1

When I'm thinking up new recipes, I'm always asking myself the same two questions: Is it going to fill me up? And is it something I want to eat? This super-quick and simple bowl has me at yes and yes. Chickpeas and avocados always scratch the itch for something hearty, the rest of the ingredients are things you will most likely already have in your crisper, and the Lemon-Herb Caesar brings it all together. Especially during a busy week, you'll love reaching for this dish.

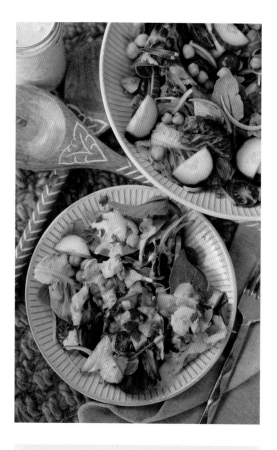

4 cups spring greens
½ **cup cherry tomatoes, halved**
½ **cup sliced English cucumber**
1 **cup canned chickpeas (164g), drained and rinsed**
½ **medium avocado (50g), peeled, pitted, and sliced**
¼ **cup red onion (from 1 small onion)**
¼ **cup fresh cilantro leaves, chopped**
6 **tablespoons Lemon-Herb Caesar (page 198)**

In a medium bowl, toss together the greens, tomatoes, cucumber, chickpeas, avocado, onion, and cilantro. Drizzle with the dressing and toss again to combine.

NOTE: You'll have about ½ cup of leftover chickpeas. You could either use them to make Simple Hummus (page 202), add them to the Breakfast Salad (page 80), or toss them with spices and bake until crisp! This salad would also be delicious with the Smokehouse Ranch (page 197).

NUTRITION FACTS
FOR 1 SERVING: CALORIES: 185 PROTEIN: 23g CARBS: 46g FAT: 22g

Japanese Nourish Bowl

SERVES
1

Kale is one of those vegetables that people either love . . . or don't. This will probably come as quite a shock, but I'm someone who used to avoid kale at all costs. Eventually, I realized I wasn't doing it any favors with how I was preparing it; it needs a little love. When sautéed until tender with onions and mushrooms and sprinkled with teriyaki coconut aminos, the greens become mild and slightly sweet and take on the flavor of all the other ingredients. Needless to say, I'm a big fan of this dish—and so are my kids! They devour their bowls every time I make them, especially if I serve them with teriyaki seaweed. My daughter makes little tacos with the seaweed, while my son likes to break it up and sprinkle it over his bowl.

Cooking spray (see page 33; optional)

5 ounces shiitake mushrooms, wiped clean, stems removed, and sliced

½ small yellow onion (110g), diced

3 tablespoons teriyaki coconut aminos

1 tablespoon minced garlic

1 teaspoon oil-free chili paste (I like sambal oelek)

½ teaspoon minced fresh ginger

2 cups chopped kale leaves (see Note)

1½ cups (237g) cooked white or brown rice

Chopped scallions (green parts only), for serving

¼ teaspoon sesame oil

Sesame seeds, for serving

Teriyaki seaweed, for serving (optional)

1. Heat a large nonstick skillet over medium heat. If you like, you can coat the pan with cooking spray to encourage even cooking, but it isn't necessary. Add the mushrooms, onion, and teriyaki coconut aminos and cook, stirring occasionally, until the mushrooms and onion are tender, about 5 minutes. If the vegetables start to stick, you can add a splash of water.

2. Add the garlic, chili paste, and ginger and cook, stirring, just until fragrant, about 2 minutes. Stir in the kale and cook until wilted and tender, about 2 minutes. Remove the pan from the heat.

3. Add the rice to a medium serving bowl and top with the kale mixture. Sprinkle with the scallions, sesame oil, and sesame seeds and enjoy with the teriyaki seaweed, if desired.

NOTE: My favorite way to chop kale leaves is to first run my knife down both sides of the rib. Then I stack the leaves in a pile and run my knife through them like a chiffonade until the kale is chopped to my liking. If you're still unconvinced about kale, you're welcome to use spinach here instead.

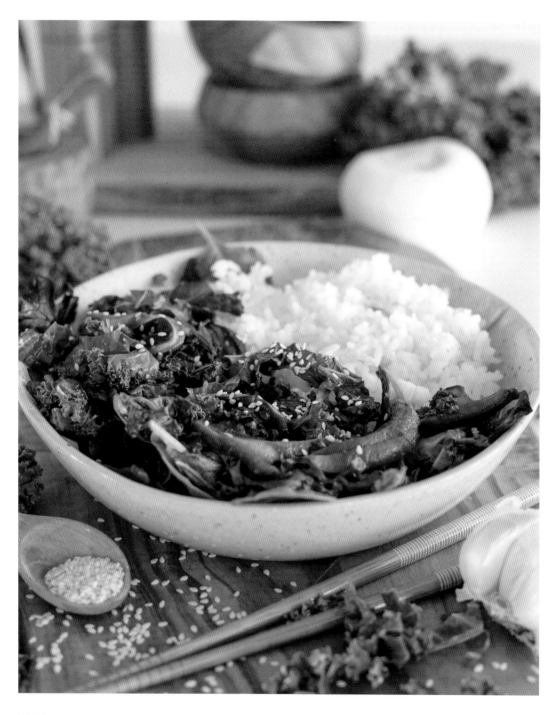

NUTRITION FACTS
FOR 1 SERVING: **CALORIES:** 443 **PROTEIN:** 12g **CARBS:** 80g **FAT:** 5g

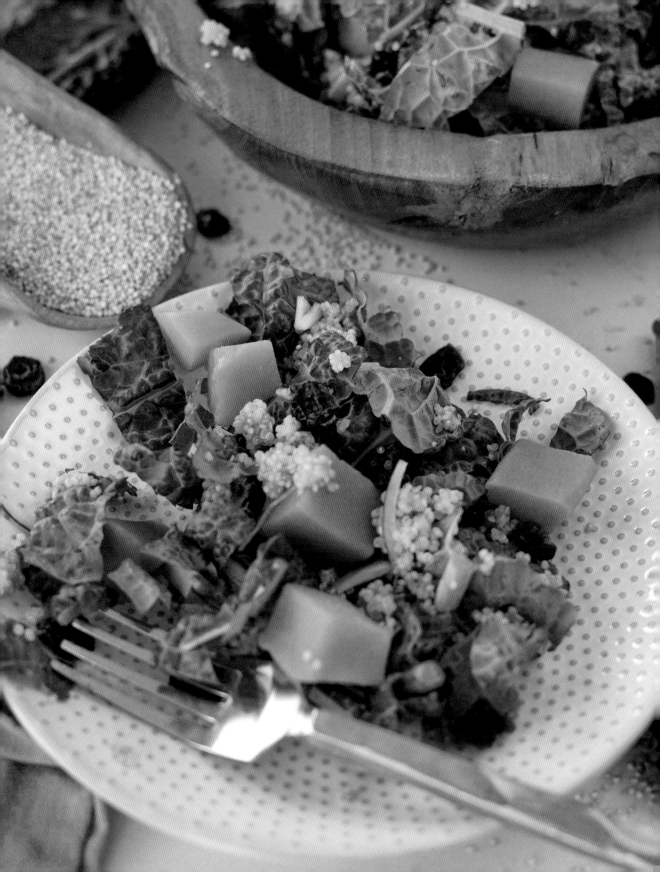

Butternut Squash and Kale Salad with Cranberries and Pecans

SERVES
1

When it comes to filling your plate with low-calorie-density foods to feel completely sated, it doesn't get much better than a salad—especially one that includes both cooked and raw veggies in addition to a grain. (Or technically a seed, in the case of quinoa.) But the real beauty of this dish is the layers of complementary flavors and textures, from the sweet and creamy squash to the earthy quinoa to the tart dried cranberries to the bright, garlicky Lemon-Herb Caesar dressing.

---

2 cups peeled and cubed butternut squash

Cooking spray (see page 33)

¼ teaspoon garlic salt

Freshly ground black pepper, to taste

1 cup water

¼ cup dry white quinoa (170g)

3 cups shredded lacinato kale leaves

2 tablespoons dried cranberries

1 tablespoon pecans, toasted in a dry pan until fragrant

¼ cup Lemon-Herb Caesar dressing (page 198)

---

1. Preheat the oven to 425°F. Line a baking sheet with parchment paper.

2. Add the squash to the baking sheet and lightly coat with cooking spray. Season with the garlic salt and a few twists of pepper and spread into a single even layer. Bake until beginning to brown, about 20 minutes.

3. Meanwhile, add the water to a medium pot and bring to a boil over medium-high heat. Add the quinoa and reduce to a simmer. Cover and cook according to the package instructions (about 15 minutes), until all the water has been absorbed. Remove the pot from the heat.

4. Add the kale, cranberries, and pecans to a large bowl. Top with the quinoa and squash, drizzle with the Lemon-Herb Caesar dressing, and toss to combine.

> **NOTE:** I like scaling up this recipe and prepping the roasted squash and quinoa at the beginning of the week so I only need to throw everything together when it's time to eat. Store the roasted squash and cooked quinoa in separate airtight containers in the refrigerator for up to 5 days.

NUTRITION FACTS

FOR 1 RECIPE: CALORIES: 482 **PROTEIN:** 14g **CARBS:** 65g **FAT:** 16g

The Preload
Soup and Salad

One of my favorite hacks for taking the edge off my appetite before a meal—which is basically insurance that I won't eat more than my body really needs at that moment—is to preload with a simple salad and/or soup. This comes in especially handy before eating out or going to a party where you don't have as much control over your food options and might feel tempted to indulge more than you'd like. These are easy to prepare and still just as delicious as the rest of your planned meal.

Preload Soup

2 medium Roma tomatoes, chopped
1 cup chopped zucchini
1 cup chopped baby bella mushrooms
½ cup diced white onion
1 tablespoon tomato paste
1 to 2 vegetable bouillon cubes (see page 33)
2 teaspoons minced garlic
½ teaspoon Italian seasoning
Sea salt and freshly ground black pepper, to taste
3 cups water

In a medium pot, combine the tomatoes, zucchini, mushrooms, onion, tomato paste, bouillon cubes, garlic, and Italian seasoning with a pinch of salt and a couple of twists of black pepper. Add the water and bring to a simmer over medium heat. Continue simmering until the veggies are tender and the flavors have melded, 12 to 15 minutes.

Preload Salad

4 cups of your favorite greens
1 cup chopped nonstarchy veggies of your choice (such as cucumbers, onion, tomato, olives, artichokes, or mushrooms)
Dressing of your choice from pages 194–201

In a large bowl, combine the greens and veggies and drizzle with the dressing. Toss well and enjoy!

NUTRITION FACTS
FOR 1 SOUP RECIPE: CALORIES: 109 PROTEIN: 7g CARBS: 11g FAT: 4g
FOR 1 SALAD RECIPE, NOT INCLUDING DRESSING: CALORIES: 57 PROTEIN: 3g CARBS: 6g FAT: 2g

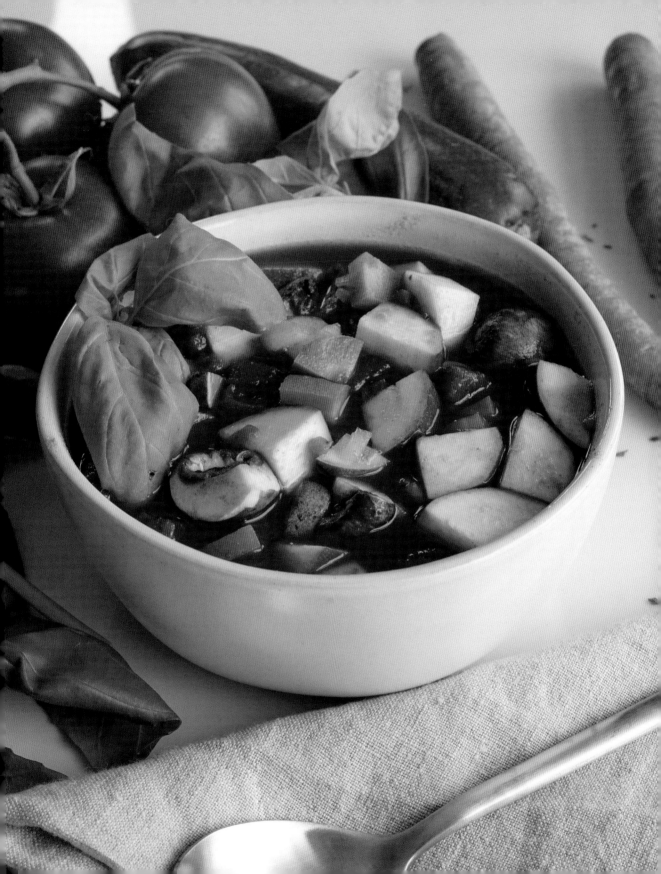

CHAPTER 9

Sauces, Dressings, and Dips

You know how you've heard a million times that there's no magic spell for hitting your weight-loss goals? That you can't just wave a wand and watch the pounds melt away? Well, while I can't *technically* claim to possess those powers either, I can tell you that the recipes in this chapter are a pretty close second. Making a healthful meal requires virtually no effort when all you need to do is keep a few of these condiments in the fridge (I like prepping mine on Sunday night) and use them to dress up a simple baked potato, a pile of greens, some steamed veggies, a bowl of grains, or all of the above. These recipes will also help you avoid feeling like you're suffering or deprived, knowing that you can have a zippy, tangy, spicy, creamy, or saucy treat anytime you want. And that's just about as magical as it gets.

If you're following one of the meal plans on pages 47–50 or 53–56, know that many of these sauces and condiments will show up as part of the recommended recipes. I recommend making a double or even triple batch of any you particularly enjoy to keep in the fridge. You'll find storage information in each of the recipes in this chapter.

Making the Most of
Your Sauces and Condiments

The recipes in this chapter are designed to be multipurpose and are meant to turn simple ingredients into extremely quick, extremely tasty snacks and meals. I've included more ideas within each recipe; here are some to get you started:

Dunk raw veggies (think carrots, bell peppers, sugar snap peas, jicama, or cucumbers) and make it a snack or a side

Smear on bread, pita, or a wrap (see pages 33–4) and make it a snack or a sandwich (or a wrap)

Dollop on grains and greens and make it a salad or bowl

Drizzle over a baked potato and your favorite cooked veggies and make it a main dish

Toss with pasta or noodles for an instant comfort-food meal

Slather over tofu or seitan and veggies as a marinade, cook, and make it lunch or dinner

All-Purpose Asian Dressing

MAKES ABOUT
3/4
CUP

This Asian-inspired dressing has the classic combi-nation of garlic, ginger, and toasted sesame, plus a bright, tangy punch of flavor from soy sauce and lime and a kick of chili heat. I love using it as a dip-ping sauce with Asian-Inspired Vegetable Pan-cakes (page 100), but it would also be great with any rice or noodle dish or a stir-fry.

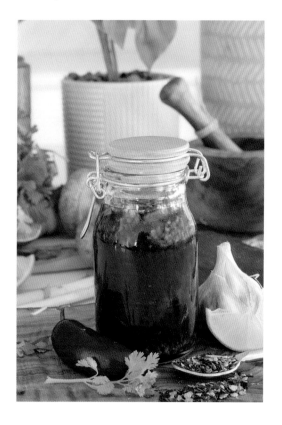

¼ cup low-sodium soy sauce

3 tablespoons fresh lime juice

3 tablespoons water

1 small shallot, minced

2 teaspoons chili paste (see page 177)

1 teaspoon minced garlic

½ teaspoon toasted sesame oil

½ teaspoon minced ginger or
¼ teaspoon ground ginger

Pinch of chili flakes

3 to 4 drops of stevia or monk fruit sweetener

1. In a medium bowl, whisk together the soy sauce, lime juice, water, shallot, chili paste, garlic, ses-ame oil, ginger, and chili flakes. Adjust the flavor as desired with stevia or monk fruit sweetener.

2. Store in a sealed jar or container in the refrig-erator for up to 5 days.

NUTRITION FACTS
FOR 1 TABLESPOON: CALORIES: 7   PROTEIN: 1g   CARBS: 1g   FAT: 0g

Creamy Sriracha Dressing

MAKES ABOUT
3/4
CUP

Blended cashews are the secret to this creamy dressing, which gets a major dose of flavor from sriracha. This one pairs particularly nicely with Asian-inspired recipes, whether a rice bowl, noodle dish, or stir-fry. But I've also been known to drizzle it over tacos!

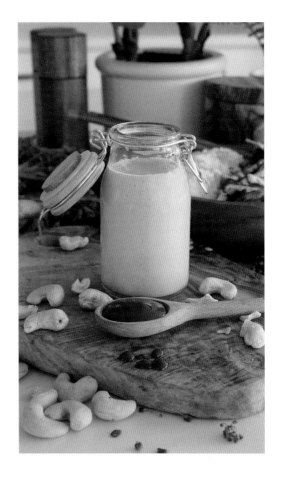

½ cup raw cashews

½ cup plain, unsweetened almond milk

1 tablespoon sriracha, plus more to taste

1 teaspoon rice vinegar

½ teaspoon sea salt

¼ teaspoon garlic powder

⅛ teaspoon toasted sesame oil

1. In a blender, combine the cashews, almond milk, sriracha, rice vinegar, salt, garlic powder, and toasted sesame oil and blend until smooth. Add more sriracha, if desired.

2. Store in a sealed jar or container in the refrigerator for up to 1 week.

NUTRITION FACTS
FOR 1 TABLESPOON: CALORIES: 12   PROTEIN: 0.3g   CARBS: 2g   FAT: 0.4g

Pesto Dressing

This is just what it sounds like—a tasty dressing that combines the fresh, herbaceous flavors of pesto with a thick, creamy sauce. I especially love it with my Pesto Pasta Primavera (page 162) and as a spread on sandwiches and wraps.

½ cup plain, unsweetened almond milk
½ cup packed fresh basil
2 tablespoons raw cashews
1 tablespoon fresh lemon juice
¼ teaspoon garlic powder
⅛ teaspoon sea salt, plus more to taste

1. In a blender, combine the almond milk, basil, cashews, lemon juice, garlic powder, and salt. Blend until smooth and season with more salt, if desired.

2. Store in a sealed jar or container in the refrigerator for up to 5 days.

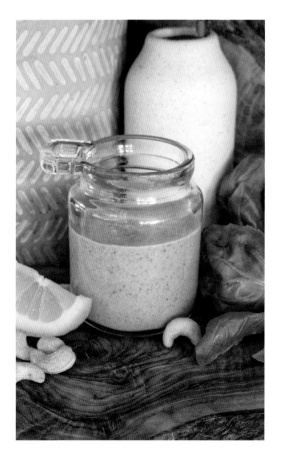

NUTRITION FACTS
FOR ⅓ CUP: **CALORIES:** 60 **PROTEIN:** 2g **CARBS:** 3g **FAT:** 4g

Smokehouse Ranch

I don't think I need to sell you on having more ranch dressing in your life. This version gets tons of flavor from herbs and spices, with no high-fat dairy or sugar required! Use this anytime you'd normally reach for your favorite dressing to dip and drizzle—or for more inspo, check out my Saucy Portobello Sammies (page 129), Herby White Bean Sammy (page 124), Hawaiian Street Cart Tacos (page 137), and Fajita Bowl (page 184).

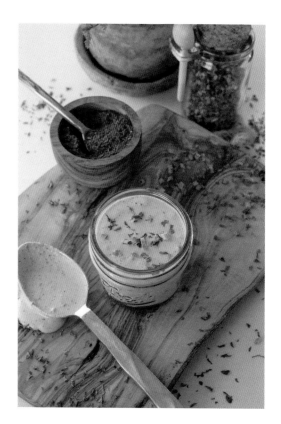

1 cup plain, unsweetened almond milk

¾ cup raw cashews

1 tablespoon distilled white vinegar

1 tablespoon ketchup

½ teaspoon smoked paprika

¼ teaspoon garlic powder

⅛ teaspoon onion powder

⅛ teaspoon chipotle powder

3 drops stevia sweetener

1 tablespoon dried chives

1 tablespoon dried parsley

1. In a blender, combine the almond milk, cashews, vinegar, ketchup, smoked paprika, garlic powder, onion powder, chipotle powder, and stevia. Blend until smooth. Use a spoon or spatula to fold in the chives and parsley.

2. Store in a sealed container in the refrigerator for up to 5 days.

NUTRITION FACTS
FOR 1 TABLESPOON: CALORIES: 27 PROTEIN: 1g CARBS: 2g FAT: 2g

Lemon-Herb Caesar

MAKES

1¾

CUPS

I've taken everything you love about a classic Cae-sar dressing—the creaminess, the savory-ness, the just-the-right saltiness—and given it a plant-based makeover. Plus I added a big hit of lemon for an extra-bright punch that wakes up any dish. Let your imagination run wild when thinking about where to drizzle and spread this dressing, but my favorites are my Mushroom Steak and "Eggs" with Herby Caesar (page 97), Garlic Herb Potato Waffles (page 102), and Chickpea Avocado Bowl (page 185). Hungry yet?

1 cup plain, unsweetened almond milk

¾ cup raw cashews

2 tablespoons fresh lemon juice

2 teaspoons brine-packed capers, drained, plus 3 teaspoons caper brine

2 teaspoons Dijon mustard

½ teaspoon sea salt, plus more to taste

¼ teaspoon garlic powder

⅛ teaspoon onion powder

Freshly ground black pepper, to taste

2 tablespoons dried chives

1 tablespoon dried parsley

1. In a blender, combine the almond milk, cashews, lemon juice, capers and brine, Dijon, salt, garlic powder, onion powder, and a few twists of black pepper. Blend until smooth. Use a spoon or spat-ula to fold in the herbs and season with more salt and pepper, if desired.

2. Store in a sealed container in the refrigerator for up to 5 days.

NUTRITION FACTS

FOR 1 TABLESPOON: **CALORIES:** 22 **PROTEIN:** 1g **CARBS:** 1g **FAT:** 2g

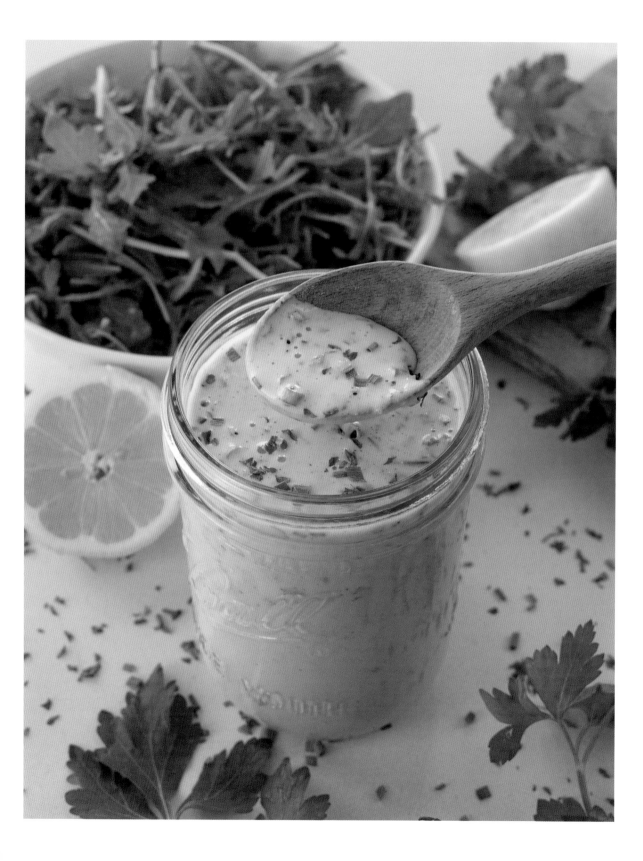

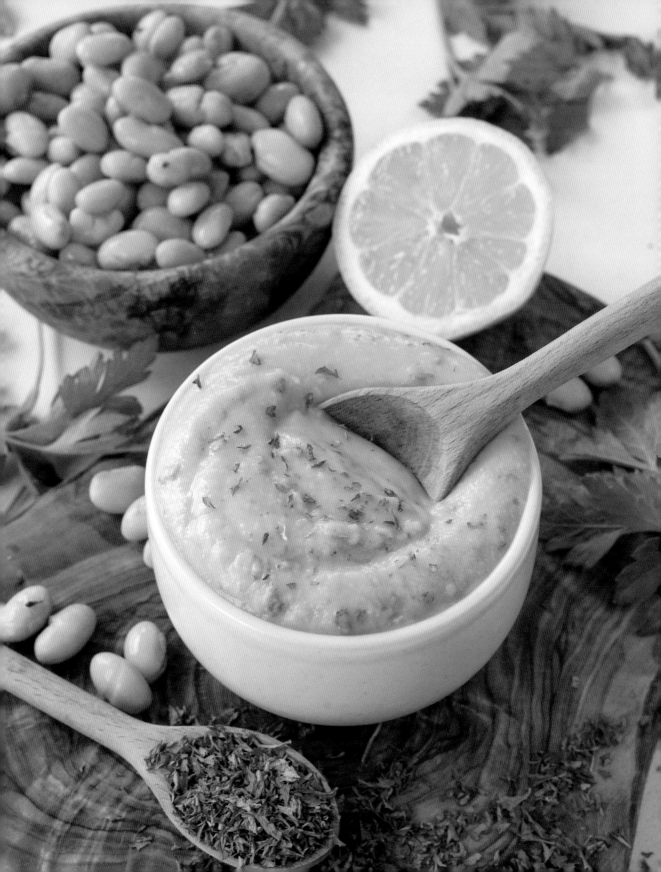

Lemony White Bean Dressing

MAKES
1½
CUPS

Protein-rich, mild-tasting white beans that puree into the creamiest spreads and dressings are the secret to low-fat, plant-based eating that's never boring. You can dress them up with pretty much any of your favorite flavors, which for me means bright notes of lemon and Dijon. You can also add a smoky kick by sprinkling in some smoked paprika. Try this with my Garlic Herb Potato Waffles (page 102) for a savory breakfast.

1 (15-ounce) can Great Northern
white beans, drained and rinsed

¼ cup water

2 tablespoons fresh lemon juice

1 tablespoon Dijon mustard

1 tablespoon maple syrup

½ teaspoon garlic powder

½ teaspoon smoked paprika (optional)

¼ teaspoon onion powder

¼ teaspoon sea salt, plus more to taste

Freshly ground black pepper, to taste

1 tablespoon dried parsley

1. In a blender, combine the beans, water, lemon juice, Dijon, maple syrup, garlic powder, smoked paprika (if using), onion powder, and salt. Add a couple of twists of black pepper and blend until smooth. Use a spoon or spatula to fold in the parsley and season with more salt, if desired.

2. Store in a sealed container in the refrigerator for up to 5 days.

NUTRITION FACTS
FOR 1 TABLESPOON: CALORIES: 20   PROTEIN: 1g   CARBS: 3g   FAT: 0g

Simple Hummus

MAKES
1
CUP

I always have hummus on hand. It's the easiest way to add extra body and richness to a bowl, salad, or sandwich; it works as a sandwich spread and a dip; it's the perfect energy-fueling snack with raw veggies or a low-calorie pita. This recipe makes sure you can reach for hummus whenever you want, because it doesn't have the oil that more traditional versions call for.

---

1 (15-ounce) can chickpeas, drained and rinsed

¼ cup water

1 tablespoon fresh lemon juice

½ tablespoon tahini paste

½ teaspoon sea salt

¼ teaspoon garlic powder

⅛ teaspoon ground cumin

---

1. In a blender, combine the chickpeas, water, lemon juice, tahini paste, salt, garlic powder, and cumin. Blend until smooth.

2. Store in a sealed container in the refrigerator for up to 1 week.

NOTE: This is a great recipe for playing around with your favorite flavors. You could add a little garlic or jalapeño (about a teaspoon will do the trick), a small handful of fresh herbs, or a pinch of curry powder or smoked paprika.

NUTRITION FACTS
FOR ¼ CUP: **CALORIES:** 99 **PROTEIN:** 5g **CARBS:** 10g **FAT:** 3g

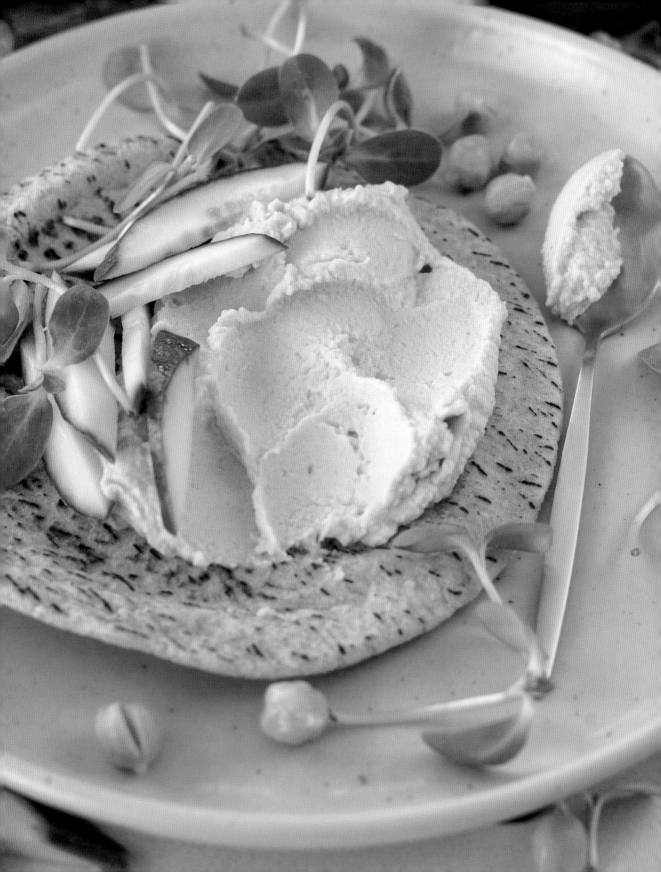

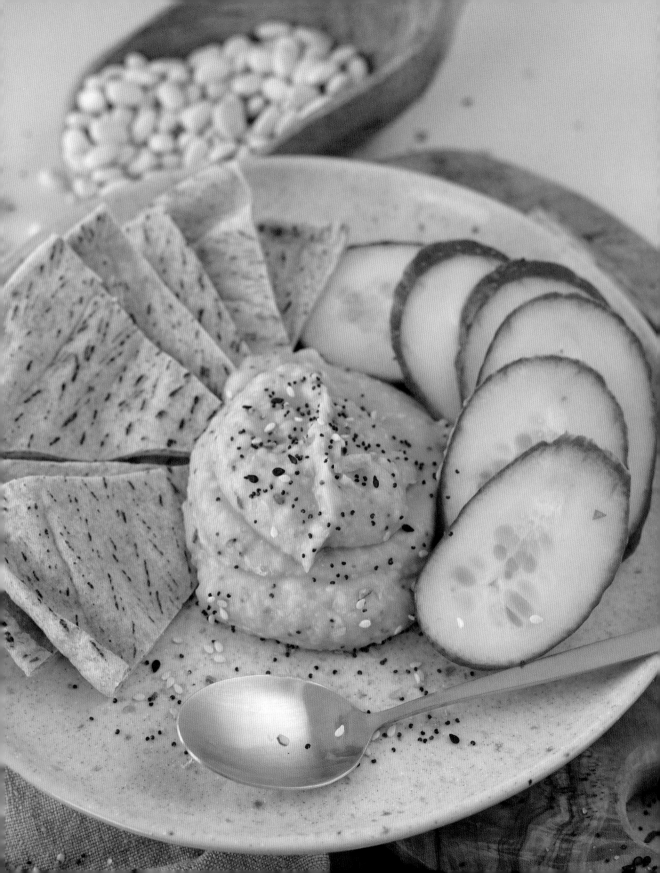

Everything Bagel
Bean Dip

MAKES

1¼

CUPS

This creamy dip gets big, bold flavor from store-bought everything bagel seasoning, which typically includes dried onion and garlic plus plenty of poppy and sesame seeds. It's a kitchen staple for me, because with a batch waiting in the fridge, I know that I can have a high-protein, low-fat snack or meal fix whenever I need it.

1. In a blender, combine the beans, water, lemon juice, Dijon, maple syrup, and garlic powder. Blend until smooth, then use a spoon or spatula to fold in the everything bagel seasoning.

2. Store in a sealed container in the refrigerator for up to 1 week.

---

1 (15-ounce) can Great Northern white beans, drained and rinsed

¼ cup water

1 tablespoon fresh lemon juice

½ tablespoon Dijon mustard

1 teaspoon maple syrup

¼ teaspoon garlic powder

1 tablespoon everything bagel seasoning

NUTRITION FACTS
FOR ¼ CUP: **CALORIES:** 92 **PROTEIN:** 5g **CARBS:** 12g **FAT:** 0.3g

Herby Bean Dip

MAKES

1¼

CUPS

Fresh or dried herbs plus white beans is a magical combination when it comes to making a hearty condiment that also tastes and feels light. I love using this as a spread for sandwiches (check out my Herby White Bean Sammy on page 124), but there's no limit to the ways you can transform your favorite veggies and starches into delicious snacks and meals.

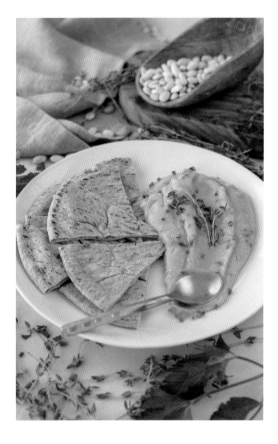

1 (15-ounce) can Great Northern
white beans, drained and rinsed

¼ cup water

1 tablespoon fresh lemon juice

½ teaspoon garlic powder

¼ teaspoon sea salt

¼ teaspoon onion powder

1 tablespoon chopped fresh or dried chives

1 tablespoon chopped fresh or dried parsley

½ tablespoon fresh thyme or
¼ teaspoon dried thyme

Freshly ground black pepper, to taste

1. In a blender, combine the beans, water, lemon juice, garlic powder, salt, and onion powder. Blend until smooth. Use a spoon or spatula to fold in the herbs and pepper.

2. Store in a sealed container in the fridge for up to 1 week.

NUTRITION FACTS
FOR ¼ CUP: **CALORIES:** 77 **PROTEIN:** 5g **CARBS:** 10g **FAT:** 0.2g

Corn and Cucumber Salsa

MAKES
3
CUPS

I used to love chips and salsa. When I chose to give up fried and processed foods, I worried that I would miss my favorite snack. I'm so happy I was wrong about that. This twist on a classic Pico de Gallo (which I've also included on page 207) has that same great, fresh flavor from cucumber and corn, plus extra-creamy texture and body from avocado. There's nothing better than a bowl of this with some cucumber slices or pita bread. It would also be great scooped onto a taco or taco bowl. I'm so glad I didn't have to break up with my favorite snack.

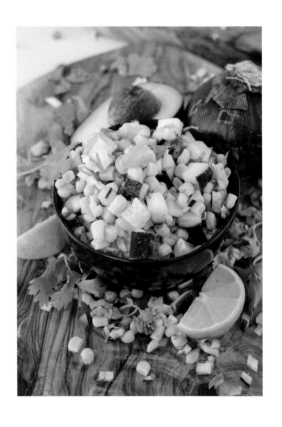

1 (15-ounce) can corn, drained

1 cup diced English cucumber

½ medium avocado (55g), diced

¼ cup chopped red onion

¼ cup chopped fresh cilantro leaves

Juice of 1 lime

¼ teaspoon sea salt, plus more to taste

⅛ teaspoon garlic powder

1. In a medium bowl, combine the corn, cucumber, avocado, onion, cilantro, lime juice, salt, and garlic powder. Give everything a gentle toss and season with more salt, if desired.

2. Store in a sealed container in the refrigerator for up to 4 days.

NUTRITION FACTS
FOR ½ CUP: CALORIES: 52 **PROTEIN:** 1g **CARBS:** 7g **FAT:** 2g

Pico de Gallo

MAKES

2

CUPS

*This is that super-fresh salsa that you frequently
see paired with Mexican dishes, the one with bite-
sized bits of tomatoes and onion flecked with
cilantro. Even before I transitioned to a low-fat,
plant-based diet, I loved adding this condiment
to my meals because of how it lifted up all the
other flavors. Now it's one of my favorite recipes
to make—and a staple of my 28-Day Meal Plans
(pages 47–50 or 53–56) because it's so simple to
assemble and so versatile for dipping and scoop-
ing—though I'm particularly partial to heaping it
over a Loaded Taco Sweet Potato (page 142).*

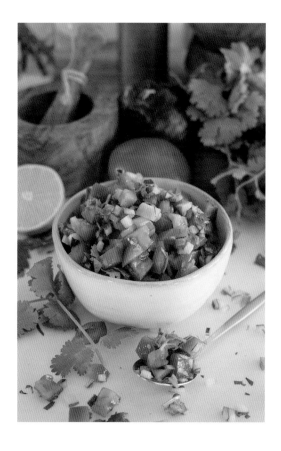

1½ cups diced Roma tomatoes
(about 3 medium tomatoes)
⅓ cup chopped fresh cilantro leaves
¼ cup diced red onion
2 tablespoons fresh lime juice
⅛ teaspoon sea salt, plus more to taste

1. In a medium bowl, combine the tomatoes, cilan-
    tro, onion, lime juice, and salt. Give everything a
    gentle toss and season with more salt, if desired.

2. Store in a sealed container in the refrigerator
    for up to 4 days.

NUTRITION FACTS
FOR ½ CUP: **CALORIES:** 21 **PROTEIN:** 1g **CARBS:** 4g **FAT:** 0g

Mango Salsa

As you can most likely tell, I love salsa. What makes this version so fun is the combination of traditional ingredients like avocado, jalapeño, and cilantro with sweet, juicy mango. The result is a refreshing condiment or dip that I'm always reaching for, especially when I want to bring sunny tropical vibes to a dish (like in the dead of winter).

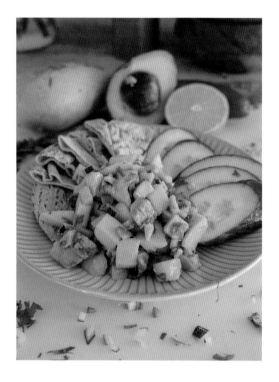

½ cup diced mango
½ medium avocado (55g), pitted, peeled, and diced
1 tablespoon minced red onion
1 tablespoon diced jalapeño
1 tablespoon chopped fresh cilantro
1 tablespoon fresh lime juice
⅛ teaspoon sea salt

1. In a medium bowl, combine the mango, avocado, onion, jalapeño, cilantro, lime juice, and salt. Give everything a gentle toss and season with more salt, if desired.

2. Store in a sealed container in the refrigerator for up to 4 days.

NUTRITION FACTS
FOR ¾ CUP: CALORIES: 182   PROTEIN: 3g   CARBS: 21g   FAT: 9g

Summer Guac

MAKES

1¼

CUPS

If there's any part of you that's not sure you could stick to a plant-based diet, just remember: Guacamole is all plants! Just like avocado makes pretty much any dish better, so does a scoop of this classic guac that I've bulked up with onions and tomatoes. It's great in all the ways you'd expect guacamole to be (on a sandwich, as a dip), but also on a Loaded Taco Sweet Potato (page 142).

2 medium avocados (210g), pitted and peeled

¼ cup diced Roma tomato (about 1 medium tomato)

¼ cup chopped fresh cilantro leaves

2 tablespoons minced red onion

2 tablespoons diced jalapeño

2 tablespoons fresh lime juice

¼ teaspoon sea salt, plus more to taste

1. In a medium bowl, use a fork to smash the avocado (make it as chunky or smooth as you like). Add the tomato, cilantro, onion, jalapeño, lime juice, and salt. Gently toss everything together and season with more salt, if desired.

2. Store in a sealed container in the refrigerator for up to 4 days.

NUTRITION FACTS

FOR ¼ CUP: CALORIES: 82   PROTEIN: 1g   CARBS: 3g   FAT: 7g

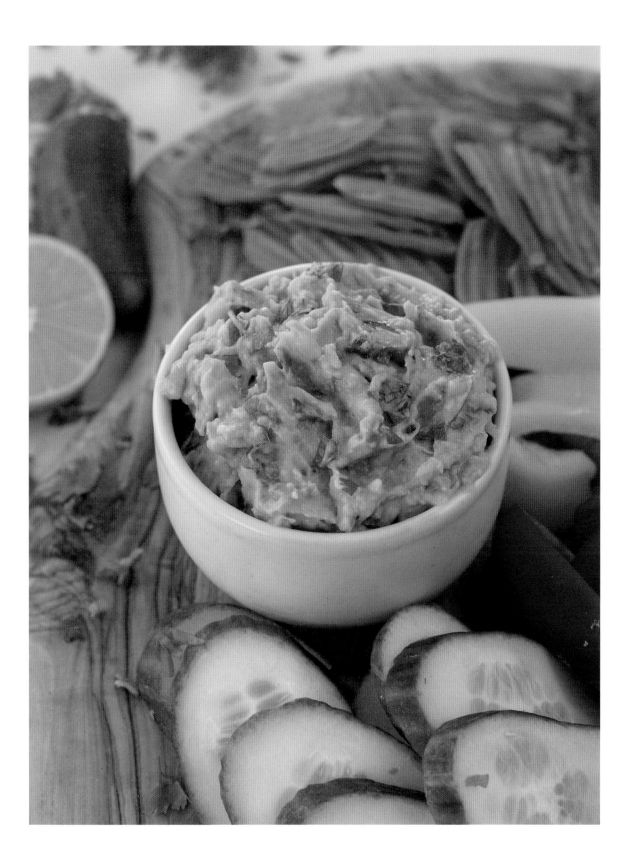

Teriyaki Sauce

MAKES

1⅓

CUPS

As a lover of teriyaki anything (noodles, rice, veg-gies, my Teriyaki Bowl on page 180), I always keep a batch of this sauce handy. It's salty-sweet and thick enough to cling to whatever you decide to toss it with, including tofu and veggies as a marinade. I especially love it on rice with my veggies!

2 tablespoons cornstarch

½ cup low-sodium soy sauce

½ cup water

½ teaspoon minced garlic or
¼ teaspoon garlic powder

¼ teaspoon minced fresh ginger or
⅛ teaspoon powdered ginger

¼ cup maple syrup

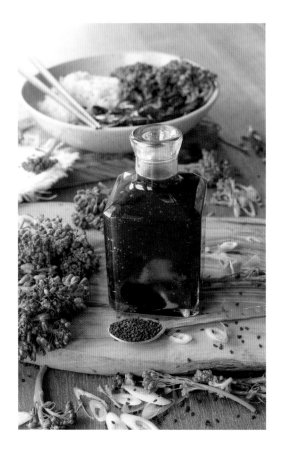

1. In a small bowl, stir together the cornstarch and ¼ cup of cold water. Set aside.

2. In a medium pot, combine the soy sauce, water, garlic, and ginger. Bring the mixture to a sim-mer, stirring occasionally, over medium-high heat. Stir in the cornstarch mixture and con-tinue stirring until the sauce thickens, about 1 minute. Turn off the heat and stir in the maple syrup.

3. Store the sauce in a sealed jar or container in the refrigerator for up to 1 week.

NUTRITION FACTS
FOR 1 TABLESPOON: **CALORIES:** 17 **PROTEIN:** 1g **CARBS:** 4g **FAT:** 0g

Roasted Red Pepper Sauce

Cashews and potatoes are what give this sauce lots of creamy body without adding significant fat or calories. When you add sun-dried tomatoes and roasted peppers to the mix, you get a velvety condiment that works well with pasta (such as my Creamy Roasted Pepper Pasta on page 165) and in bowls.

1 sun-dried tomato (not oil-packed)

½ cup peeled and diced Russet potatoes (132g)

¼ cup roasted bell peppers packed in water

2 tablespoons raw cashews

1 tablespoon liquid from roasted
bell pepper jar or water

1 teaspoon fresh lemon juice

½ teaspoon garlic powder

½ teaspoon sea salt

¼ teaspoon onion powder

1. In a small bowl, submerge the sun-dried tomato in hot water. Set aside.

2. In a small pot, combine the potatoes with just enough cold water to cover them by 1 inch. Bring to a boil over medium-high heat, reduce to a simmer, and cook, uncovered, until the potatoes are fork tender, about 15 minutes. Reserve ½ cup of the cooking water, then strain the potatoes in a colander. Remove the sun-dried tomato from the water.

3. In a blender, combine the cooked potatoes, reserved water, soaked sun-dried tomato, roasted peppers, cashews, roasted pepper liquid, lemon juice, garlic powder, salt, and onion powder. Blend until smooth.

4. Store the sauce in a sealed jar or container in the refrigerator for up to 3 days.

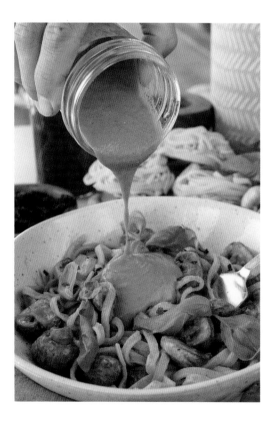

NUTRITION FACTS

FOR ¼ CUP: **CALORIES:** 45 **PROTEIN:** 1g **CARBS:** 6g **FAT:** 2g

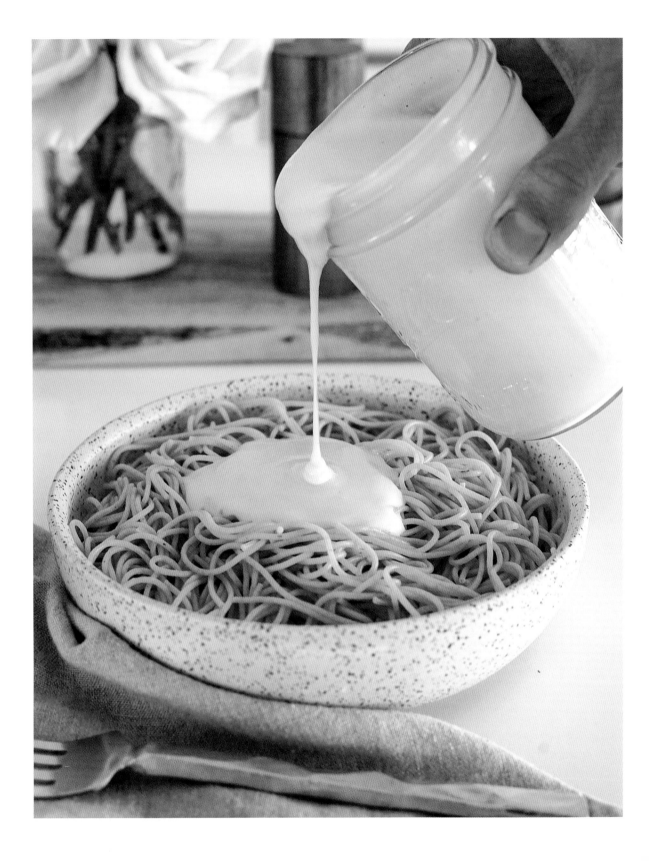

Garlic Alfredo Sauce

MAKES

2¼

CUPS

It's true—you can stick to your goals and slather your meals in a decadently rich and garlicky alfredo sauce. Of course, that's because my version doesn't involve any heavy cream. Instead, I look to potatoes and cashews to provide that luscious texture—and you'd never notice the difference! Try this on Spinach and Artichoke–Stuffed Mushrooms (page 144), Spring Alfredo Pasta (page 166), or any dish that could use the alfredo treatment.

1½ cups peeled and diced Russet potatoes (225g)

2 teaspoons garlic powder

1 teaspoon sea salt

1 teaspoon fresh lemon juice

½ teaspoon onion powder

¼ cup raw cashews

⅛ teaspoon freshly ground black pepper

1. Add the potatoes and enough cold water to cover them by 1 inch to a small pot. Bring to a boil over medium-high heat, reduce to a simmer, and cook until fork tender, about 15 minutes. Reserve 1 cup of the cooking water, then drain the potatoes in a colander.

2. In a blender, combine the cooked potatoes, reserved cooking water, garlic powder, salt, lemon juice, onion powder, cashews, and pepper. Blend until smooth.

3. Store in a sealed container in the refrigerator for up to 1 week. To reheat, microwave at 30-second intervals, stirring between each, until warmed to your liking.

NUTRITION FACTS
FOR ¼ CUP: CALORIES: 40 PROTEIN: 1g CARBS: 5g FAT: 2g

Poblano Cheese Sauce

MAKES
2¼
CUPS

Poblano peppers are one of my favorite ingredients. They have a subtle heat and a naturally smoky flavor, which really comes out when they're roasted. Blended with cashews and potatoes, they transform into a rich, flavor-packed drizzle that you can use on pretty much anything. It's the secret sauce that makes some of my favorite recipes so great: Grilled "Steak" and Cheese Sammy (page 133), Loaded Taco Sweet Potato (page 142), Cilantro-Lime Stuffed Peppers (page 157), Mexican Hash Brown Bake (page 158), and Cheesy Poblano Enchiladas (page 161).

---

1 medium poblano pepper (see Note)
1½ cups (225g) peeled and diced Russet potatoes
¼ cup raw cashews
1 teaspoon fresh lemon juice
1 teaspoon garlic powder
1 teaspoon sea salt
½ teaspoon onion powder

NOTE: You can substitute 4 ounces of canned fire-roasted green chilies for the roasted poblano.

1. Preheat the oven to 425°F. Line a baking sheet with parchment paper.

2. Place the poblano pepper on the prepared baking sheet and roast for 20 minutes, until nicely charred on all sides.

3. Meanwhile, make the potatoes: In a small pot, combine the potatoes with enough cold water to cover by 2 inches. Bring to a boil over medium-high heat, reduce to a simmer, and cook, uncovered, until the potatoes are fork tender, about 15 minutes. Reserve 1 cup of the cooking water, then drain the potatoes in a colander and set aside.

4. When the pepper is done roasting, immediately transfer it to a plastic zip-top bag or a bowl covered with plastic wrap and allow it to steam for 10 minutes. Remove the pepper and let it cool. Once comfortable enough to handle, use your hands to slip off the skin and scoop out the seeds (unless you want a lot more heat in your sauce!).

5. Transfer the pepper, cooked potatoes, and cooking water to a blender and add the cashews, lemon juice, garlic powder, salt, and onion powder. Blend until smooth.

6. Store in a sealed container in the refrigerator for up to 1 week. To reheat, microwave at 30-second intervals, stirring between each, until warmed to your liking.

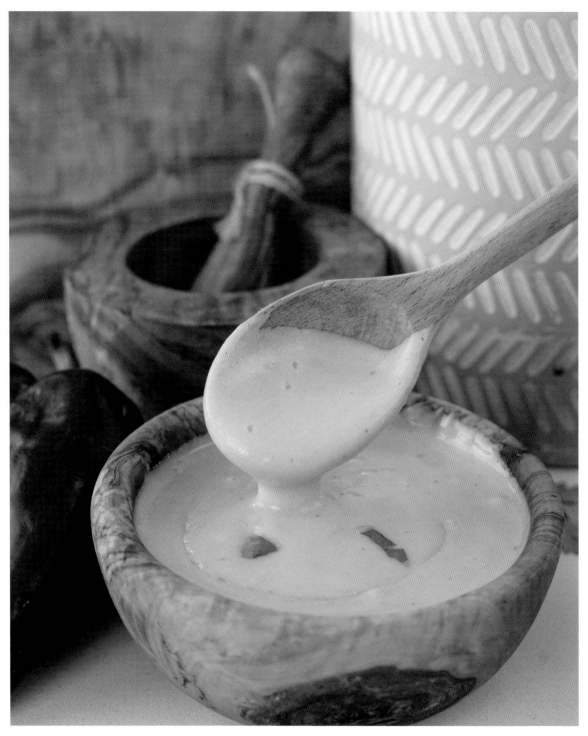

NUTRITION FACTS
FOR ¼ CUP: **CALORIES:** 43 **PROTEIN:** 1g **CARBS:** 5g **FAT:** 2g

Avocado Lime Crema

MAKES

$2\frac{1}{4}$

CUPS

I was born on the Yucatán Peninsula in Mexico, and for me, Mexican food is life. So, when I went plant-based, the dishes I figured out how to re-create first were my beloved Mexican staples. And the one condiment that's key to these dishes is cool, creamy, tangy crema. This dairy-free version is exactly that, thanks to avocado and pops of jalapeño and lime. Drizzle this over Black Bean Tacos (page 134), a Loaded Taco Sweet Potato (page 142, Cheesy Poblano Enchiladas (page 161), Smoky Sweet Chili (page 174), or any other dish that could use a little brightening up.

2 medium avocados (250g), pitted, peeled, and scooped

½ cup chopped fresh cilantro leaves

½ cup water

1 medium jalapeño, seeds removed if you prefer less heat

5 tablespoons fresh lime juice (from about 2 large limes)

¼ teaspoon sea salt

¼ teaspoon garlic powder

¼ teaspoon onion powder

1. In a blender, combine the avocados, cilantro, water, jalapeño, lime juice, salt, garlic powder, and onion powder. Blend until smooth.

2. Store in a sealed container in the refrigerator for up to 3 days.

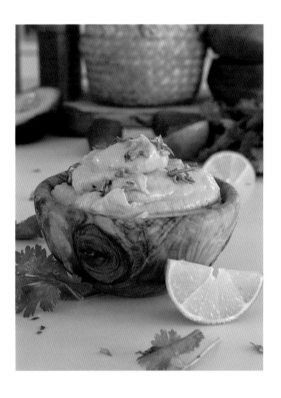

NUTRITION FACTS

FOR 1 TABLESPOON: CALORIES: 13 PROTEIN: 0g CARBS: 1g FAT: 1g

Cashew Lime Crema

This is a zesty twist on a "traditional" cashew sour cream using bright, tangy lime juice. It can be used anywhere you'd use either sour cream or crema, such as drizzled over soups or any of the tacos from pages 134–41.

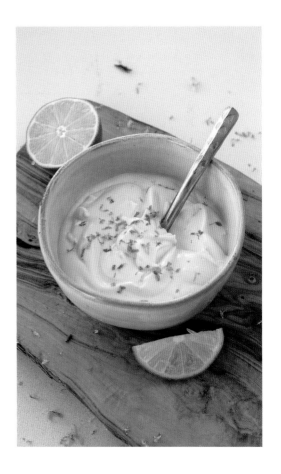

¾ cup raw cashews, soaked overnight
or boiled for 8 minutes

¼ cup water

5 teaspoons fresh lime juice

1½ teaspoons white vinegar

¼ teaspoon sea salt, plus more to taste

⅛ teaspoon garlic powder

2 drops of stevia sweetener

1. In a blender, combine the cashews, water, lime juice, vinegar, salt, garlic powder, and stevia. Blend until smooth. Season with more salt, if desired.

2. Store in a sealed container in the refrigerator for up to 5 days.

NUTRITION FACTS
FOR 1 TABLESPOON: **CALORIES:** 39 **PROTEIN:** 1g **CARBS:** 2g **FAT:** 3g

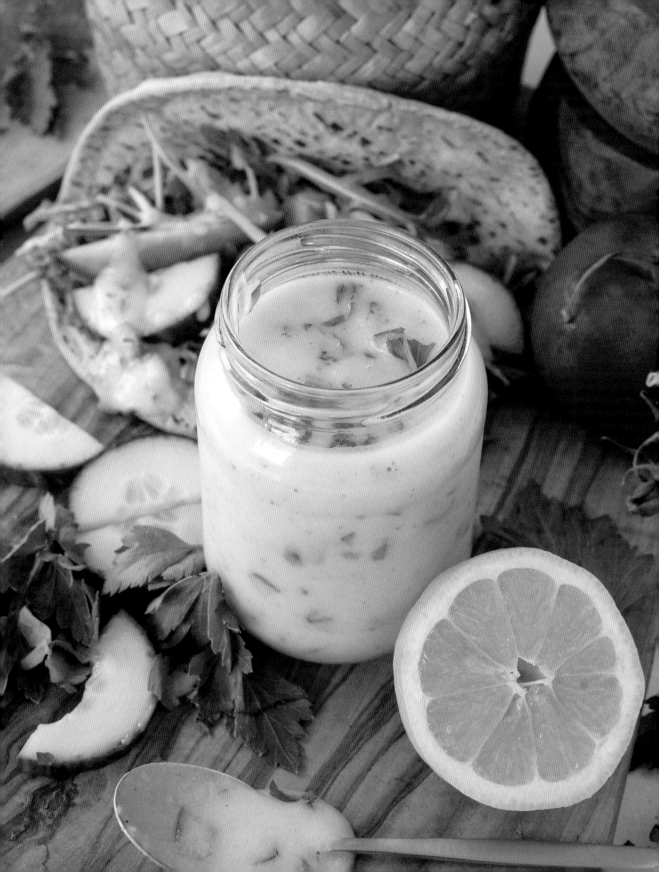

Tzatziki Sauce

MAKES

1¼

CUPS

Tzatziki is a yogurt sauce frequently served with Middle Eastern and Mediterranean dishes. Spiked with lemon juice and garlic, it offers a fresh, bright lift to pretty much any dish, but especially anything with bold spices. Try it spread over an "Egg" and Avocado Breakfast Sandwich (page 106) or drizzled over Falafel Cauliflower Pitas (page 120).

1 cup plain unsweetened coconut
yogurt (see page 34)

¼ cup chopped fresh parsley leaves

1 tablespoon fresh lemon juice

½ teaspoon minced garlic

¼ teaspoon sea salt, plus more to taste

Freshly ground black pepper, to taste

1. In a medium bowl, stir together the yogurt, parsley, lemon juice, garlic, salt, and a couple of twists of black pepper.

2. Store in a sealed container in the refrigerator for up to 5 days.

NUTRITION FACTS
FOR ¼ CUP: **CALORIES:** 24 **PROTEIN:** 0g **CARBS:** 2g **FAT:** 2g

Remoulade

MAKES

1

CUP

Remoulade, a traditional French condiment, is a great all-purpose dip-sauce hybrid that adds instant richness to a dish. It's a blend of mayo, capers, and chopped pickles, so I've simply substituted naturally creamy cashews for the mayo and subbed in relish (any brand will do!) so there's no chopping involved. The delicious sweet-sour taste is still very much the same and pairs perfectly with Vegan Crab Cakes (page 154) or makes a fantastic burger sauce or sandwich spread.

½ cup raw cashews

½ cup plain, unsweetened almond milk

2 tablespoons ketchup

2 teaspoons brined capers

2 teaspoons caper brine

1 teaspoon Dijon mustard

1 teaspoon white vinegar

½ teaspoon sea salt

¼ teaspoon garlic powder

1 tablespoon sweet relish

---

1. In a blender, combine the cashews, almond milk, ketchup, capers, caper brine, Dijon, vinegar, salt, and garlic powder. Blend until smooth. Use a spoon or spatula to fold in the relish.

2. Store in a sealed container in the refrigerator for up to 5 days.

NUTRITION FACTS

FOR 1 TABLESPOON: CALORIES: 27   PROTEIN: 1g   CARBS: 2g   FAT: 2g

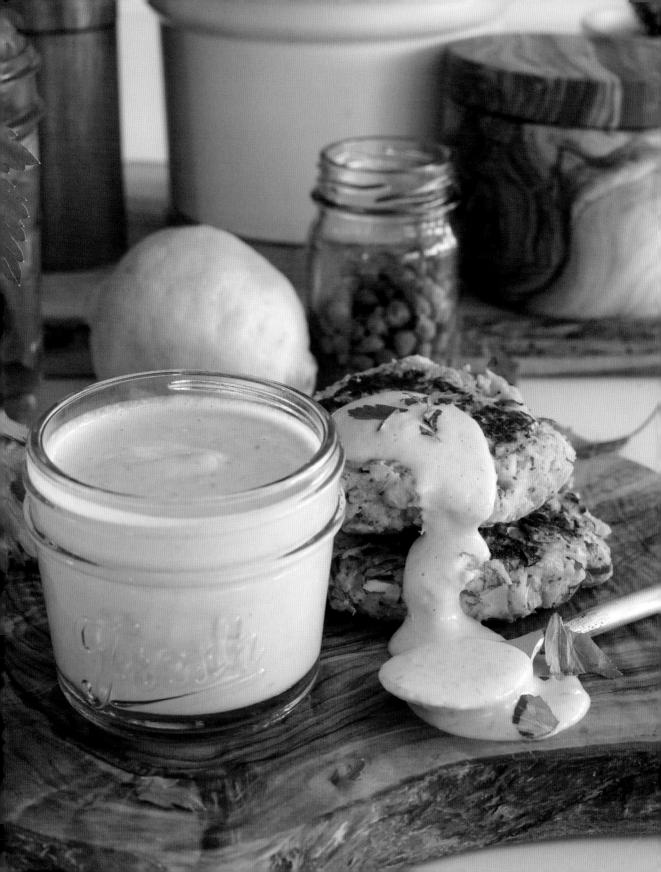

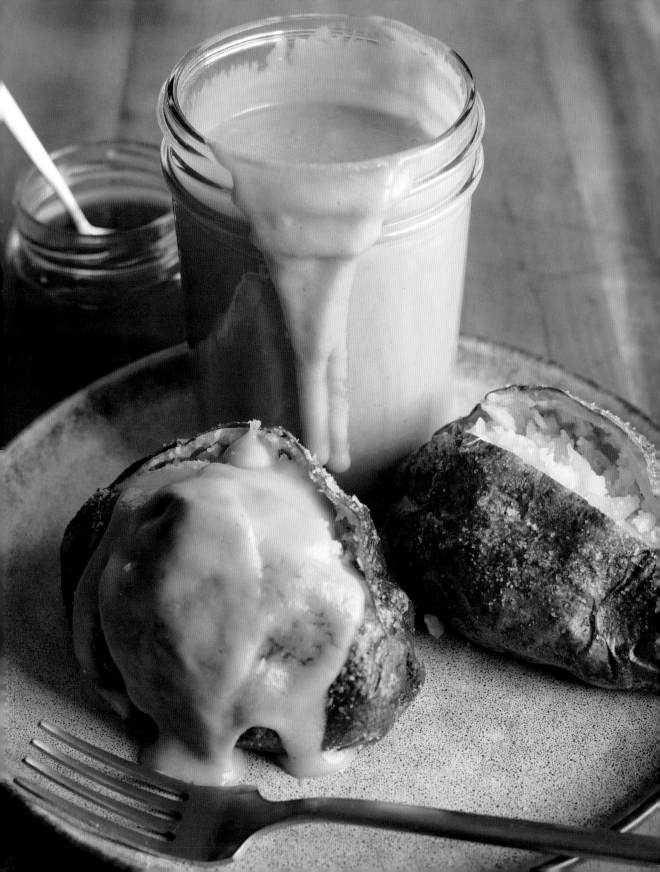

Pimento Cheese Sauce

MAKES

2½

CUPS

As a huge believer in the power of sauces to take any dish or meal to the next level, I wanted to try my hand at making a "traditional" southern pimento cheese sauce. This beloved condiment normally gets its creaminess from a mixture of cheese and mayo, but that's not exactly what we're about here. Instead, I layered potatoes and cashews with the more typical flavor boosters such as pickled jalapeños and, of course, pimentos. Try this draped over Hawaiian Potatoes (page 171), Apple Pimento Grilled Cheese with Caramelized Onions and Arugula (page 125), or even Black Bean Tacos (page 134).

---

2 cups (275g) Yukon Gold potatoes, diced

½ cup diced carrots (about 1 large carrot)

¼ cup raw cashews

3 tablespoons chopped jarred pimentos

2 tablespoons pickled jalapeños

1 teaspoon garlic salt

1 teaspoon fresh lemon juice

1 teaspoon vegan Worcestershire sauce

¼ teaspoon onion powder

---

1. Place the potatoes in a medium pot and add just enough cold water to cover by about 1 inch. Bring to a boil over medium-high heat, reduce to a simmer, and cook until the potatoes are fork tender, 10 to 15 minutes. Reserve 1 cup of water from the pot and drain.

2. In a blender, combine the cooked potatoes, water, carrots, cashews, pimentos, jalapeños, garlic salt, lemon juice, Worcestershire sauce, and onion powder. Blend until smooth.

3. Store in a sealed container in the refrigerator for up to 5 days.

NUTRITION FACTS
FOR ¼ CUP: **CALORIES:** 41 **PROTEIN:** 1g **CARBS:** 6g **FAT:** 1g

CHAPTER 10

Desserts

As you now know, I would never deprive myself when it comes to delicious meals, and I would never want that for you, either. That's why my goal has always been to create decadent, satisfying dishes—that just so happen to feature low-fat, plant-based ingredients. The recipes in this chapter are no different. There's something for every craving—chocolatey and fruity, creamy and crunchy, cold and warm—with no limitations on how much you can enjoy them. That's because at their foundation are whole foods that deliver peak nutrition while also supporting your health and weight-loss goals. Whether you reach for these sweet treats as a snack, a midday pick-me-up, or an after-dinner nibble, you can feel good about continuing to give yourself the love and care you deserve.

Vanilla Tapioca Pudding

SERVES
1

In late fall, when the weather started to get chilly, my mom would make my brother and me this simple pudding for dessert. We'd enjoy it warm, snuggling up around the fireplace. To this day, enjoying it makes me feel cozy and cared for.

Traditionally, you'd make this dessert with eggs, milk, and sugar, but after tinkering with the recipe, I've nailed down an almost exact replica of my childhood favorite using leaner, plant-based ingredients, but still with the fun texture of classic tapioca pearls (which are made from tapioca starch). It's the kind of treat your whole family will love.

2 tablespoons tapioca pearls

¼ cup hot water

1 cup plain, unsweetened almond milk

½ teaspoon vanilla extract

Pinch of ground cinnamon

Stevia or monk fruit drops, to taste

1. In a small bowl, soak the tapioca pearls in the hot water for 10 to 15 minutes, until the pearls have absorbed all of the liquid.

2. Transfer the soaked tapioca and any water left in the bowl to a small saucepan. Stir in the almond milk and bring the mixture to a boil over medium-high heat. Reduce to a strong simmer and cook, stirring constantly, until thickened, 3 to 5 minutes. If the mixture still hasn't thickened after 5 minutes, turn the heat up a touch.

3. Remove the pot from the heat and stir in the vanilla extract, cinnamon, and sweetener to taste. Allow the pudding to cool slightly before digging in.

NUTRITION FACTS

CALORIES: 118 **PROTEIN:** 1g **CARBS:** 22g **FAT:** 2g

One-Bowl Heavenly Banana Brownies

The name of this recipe says it all. These brownies are just as rich, gooey, and chocolatey as you'd want them to be—plus they come together quickly in one bowl. But the single most exciting feature is that you can keep the leftovers in the freezer. Pull one out, pop it in the microwave for 30 to 40 seconds, and you have an on-demand, single-serving fresh-baked brownie to enjoy.

Cooking spray (see page 33)

2 medium ripe bananas (194g)

2 tablespoons maple syrup

2 tablespoons unsweetened cocoa powder

1 teaspoon vanilla extract

½ cup gluten-free oat flour or regular all-purpose flour

1 teaspoon baking powder

⅛ teaspoon sea salt

2 tablespoons dairy-free chocolate chips (see page 33)

1. Preheat the oven to 375°F. Lightly spray a loaf pan with cooking spray and set aside.

2. In a medium bowl, use a fork to mash the bananas until smooth and creamy.

3. Add the maple syrup, cocoa powder, and vanilla to the bananas and mix well until everything is fully incorporated. Stir in the oat flour, baking powder, and salt and mix until well combined.

4. Transfer the batter to the prepared pan and use a spatula to smooth the top. Sprinkle the chocolate chips evenly over the batter. Bake until the brownies have mostly set and are still slightly gooey in the center when a knife is inserted, 18 to 20 minutes. Don't overbake or the brownies will be dry.

5. Slice into 8 even pieces and enjoy. Store leftover brownies in an airtight container at room temperature for up to 3 days, or freeze for up to 2 weeks.

NUTRITION FACTS

FOR 1 SERVING (1 BROWNIE): **CALORIES:** 81 **PROTEIN:** 2g **CARBS:** 13g **FAT:** 2g

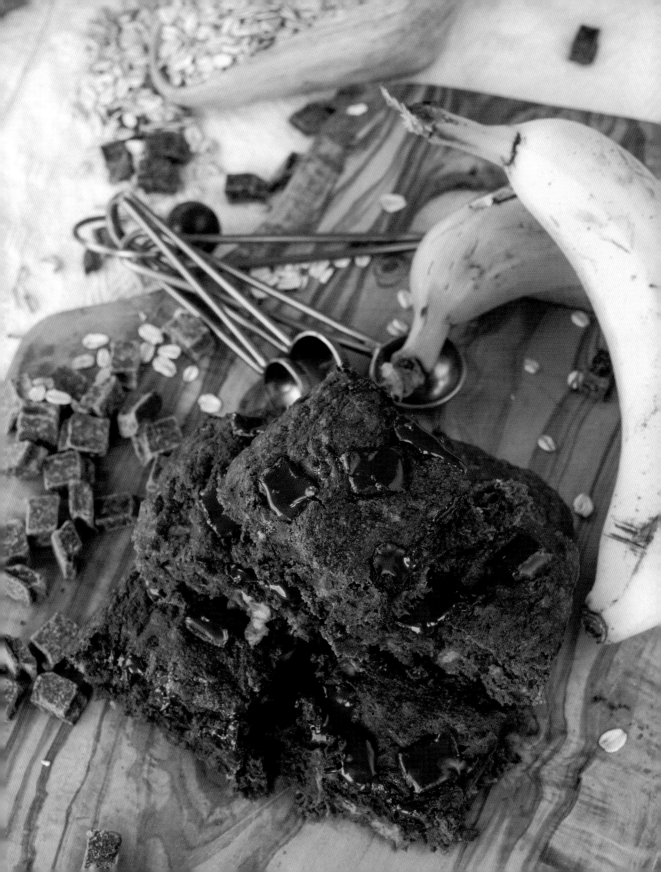

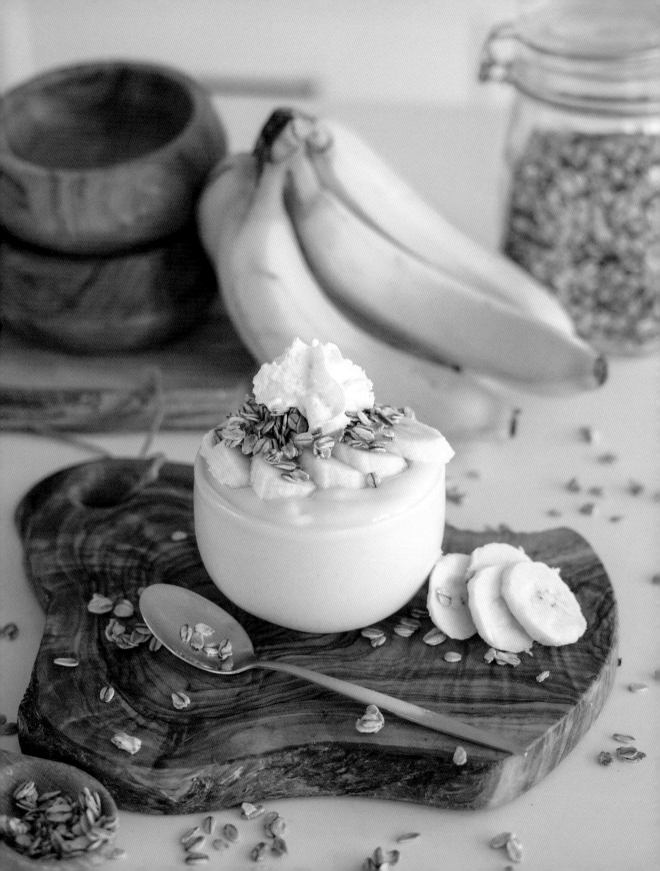

Banana Crème Pie Pudding

SERVES
1

If you love an old-school pudding pie, then this is about to be your new favorite dessert. It turns out that it's extremely easy to make luscious, creamy homemade pudding with almond milk, and you can customize it with a variety of flavors. Go classic with banana (you can find banana extract in the baking aisle of your grocery store) or switch it up with maple extract and pecans or butterscotch extract and pistachios. Whatever you decide, don't forget to finish it off with a big dollop of almond milk whipped cream. Just remember that the pudding needs 20 minutes to set if you want to enjoy it chilled.

---

1 cup plain, unsweetened almond milk

1½ tablespoons cornstarch

¼ teaspoon banana extract

¼ teaspoon vanilla extract

Stevia or monk fruit drops, to taste

½ medium banana (59g), sliced

3 tablespoons almond milk whipped cream (see page 34)

---

1. In a medium saucepan, whisk together the almond milk and cornstarch until no lumps remain. Heat the mixture over medium-high heat, whisking constantly, until it begins to boil. Reduce to a simmer and continue whisking until the mixture has thickened, about 1 minute. Remove the pan from the heat.

2. Stir in the banana and vanilla extracts and add sweetener to taste. Enjoy the pudding warm as soon as it's assembled, or allow it to chill in the refrigerator for 20 minutes. (It's best shortly after it's made.)

3. When ready to serve, top with the banana slices and whipped cream.

NUTRITION FACTS
FOR 1 SERVING: **CALORIES:** 142 **PROTEIN:** 2g **CARBS:** 28g **FAT:** 3g

Maple Pecan Pudding

Replace the banana extract with ½ teaspoon maple extract, then top the pudding with 1 tablespoon of chopped and toasted pecans instead of the sliced banana. Reduce the whipped topping to 2 tablespoons.

NUTRITION FACTS
CALORIES: 152 **PROTEIN:** 2g **CARBS:** 27g **FAT:** 4g

Strawberry Shortcake

SERVES
2
MAKES 2
SHORTCAKES

As soon as berries start popping up at the market in the spring, I begin thinking about this dessert. It's a cloudlike biscuit heaped with sweet, juicy straw-berries and whipped cream, which manages to feel both decadent and light. I love making it for com-pany, for the kids and their friends, or just myself.

---

1 cup white whole-wheat flour
1 teaspoon baking powder
⅛ teaspoon sea salt
½ cup plus 2 tablespoons water
½ teaspoon vanilla extract
1 cup hulled and chopped fresh strawberries
3 tablespoons almond milk whipped
cream (see page 34)

---

1. Preheat the oven to 375°F. Line a baking sheet with parchment paper and set aside.

2. In a small mixing bowl, whisk together the flour, baking powder, and salt until well combined.

3. In a measuring cup, stir together the water and vanilla.

4. Slowly stream the vanilla mixture into the flour mixture, whisking constantly. When the dough begins to thicken, switch to a spoon and stir until the dough is uniform.

5. Use a ½-cup measuring cup to form two evenly sized biscuits. Place them on the prepared baking sheet and bake until lightly golden, 10 to 12 minutes. Allow them to cool slightly on the pan.

6. Slice the biscuits through the middle. On the bottom half of each biscuit, mound ¼ cup of the strawberries. Set the top half of the biscuit on the berries and finish with the remaining ¼ cup strawberries and the whipped cream.

NUTRITION FACTS
FOR 1 SERVING (1 SHORTCAKE) WITH TOPPINGS: **CALORIES:** 175 **PROTEIN:** 6g **CARBS:** 30g **FAT:** 2g

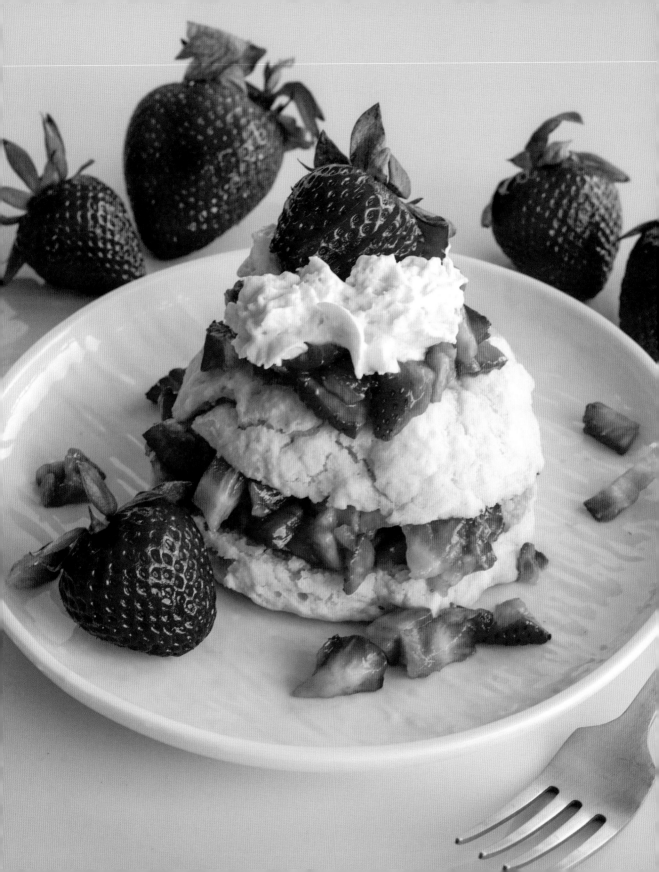

Peaches and Cream

SERVES

1

I personally think a ripe summer peach could be a dessert in its own right. But when tossed with maple syrup and cinnamon, cooked until soft and caramelized, then topped with whipped cream, it's like tucking into the best homemade peach pie you've ever tasted—and it takes all of five minutes to pull together. Don't worry, though—you don't need peaches from Colorado for this dish to be delicious.

1 large ripe peach, pitted and cut into ½-inch-thick slices

1 teaspoon fresh lemon juice

1 teaspoon maple syrup

1 teaspoon vanilla extract

Pinch of ground cinnamon

Cooking spray (see page 33)

3 tablespoons almond milk whipped cream (see page 34)

1. In a medium bowl, combine the peach slices with the lemon juice, maple syrup, vanilla, and cinnamon and toss to coat.

2. Lightly coat a large nonstick skillet with cooking spray and add the peach mixture. Cook over medium heat, stirring once or twice, until the peaches begin to soften and caramelize, about 3 minutes.

3. Transfer the peaches to a serving bowl and serve topped with the whipped cream.

NUTRITION FACTS
CALORIES: 114 PROTEIN: 2g CARBS: 20g FAT: 1g

Coffee-Chocolate Nice Cream

SERVES
1

My mom was obsessed with coffee ice cream, and, as most kids do, I would sneak spoonfuls out of the tub she always kept stashed in the freezer. Even though it wasn't like anything else I'd tasted at that point in my life, I developed a love for the coffee flavor, especially when combined with chocolate. In order to enjoy it whenever I'm in the mood, I developed this recipe, which is just as creamy, rich, and flavorful as the original I loved as a kid.

2 small bananas (200g), frozen and chopped

¼ cup plain, unsweetened almond milk

½ tablespoon instant coffee granules (I use decaf)

1 teaspoon vanilla extract

4 drops liquid stevia or monk fruit sweetener, plus more to taste

½ tablespoons dairy-free chocolate chips (see page 33)

1. In a food processor, combine the bananas, almond milk, instant coffee, vanilla, and sweetener. Process until the mixture has an ice cream–like consistency, pausing at least once to scrape down the sides of the bowl with a spatula. Taste and add more sweetener, if desired.

2. Transfer the nice cream to a serving bowl and top with the chocolate chips.

NUTRITION FACTS
CALORIES: 251 PROTEIN: 4g CARBS: 48g FAT: 4g

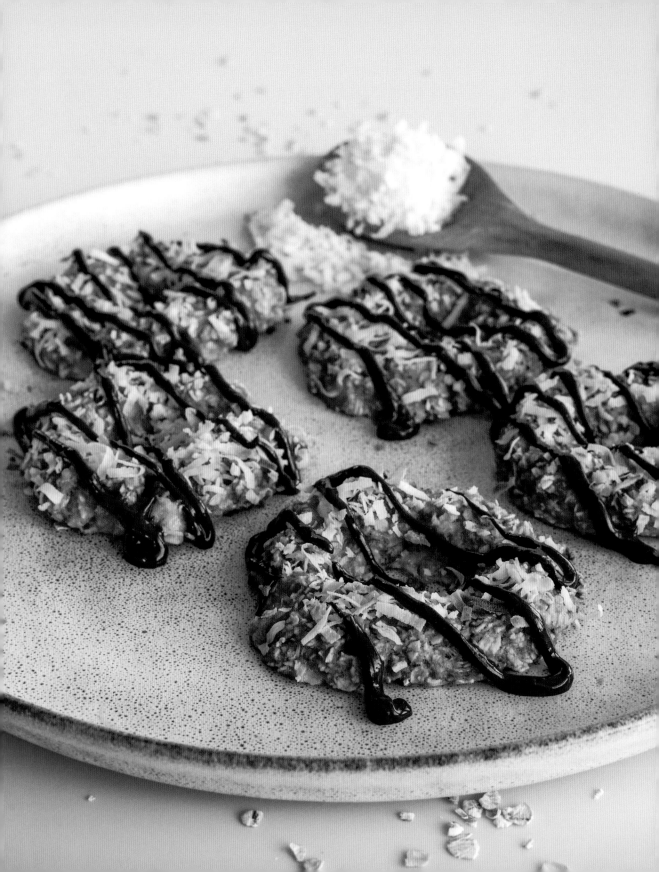

Coconut Banana Bites

SERVES
5
MAKES 5
COOKIES

I was sitting around one day thinking about how much I would enjoy a cookie with some chocolate and coconut—two of my favorite flavors—and this recipe was born. I figured out that if you bake a mashed banana and oat blend, it becomes almost cake-like. And when topped with shredded coconut and a drizzle of melted chocolate, it makes you wonder why you ever bothered with regular store-bought cookies.

---

1 large banana (118g)
1 cup rolled oats
1 teaspoon vanilla extract
1 tablespoon shredded unsweetened coconut
**2 tablespoons dairy-free chocolate
chips (see page 33)**

---

1. Preheat the oven to 375ºF. Line a baking sheet with parchment paper and set aside.

2. In a medium bowl, use a fork to mash the banana until mostly smooth. Add the oats and vanilla and stir until well incorporated.

3. Portion the mixture into 5 tablespoon-sized scoops and arrange them in a single layer on the prepared baking sheet. Use your fingers to form each scoop into a doughnut-shaped cookie. Sprinkle the cookies with the shredded coconut and bake until the coconut has begun to brown, about 10 minutes. Allow the cookies to cool slightly on the pan while you make the chocolate topping.

4. Place the chocolate chips in a small, microwave-safe bowl. Heat in 20-second increments, stirring between each, until the chocolate is melted and smooth, about 1 minute total.

5. Spoon the chocolate into a small plastic zip-top bag and snip off one corner. Pipe a drizzle of chocolate over each cookie.

6. Store leftover cookies in an airtight container at room temperature for up to 5 days, or freeze for up to 2 weeks.

NUTRITION FACTS
FOR 1 SERVING (1 COOKIE): **CALORIES:** 123 **PROTEIN:** 3g **CARBS:** 18g **FAT:** 4g

Apple Turnovers

Behold, the easiest apple turnover you could ever make, plant-based or otherwise. It requires no dough or cooking down of the filling. Rather, this gets its magic from the always-tasty combination of cinnamon and sugar, plus the surprising addition of sandwich bread. Drizzle these with a little icing and you have yourself one tasty handheld treat.

---

1 small apple (I like Honeycrisp)

1 tablespoon granulated sugar

¼ teaspoon ground cinnamon, plus more for sprinkling

2 slices sprouted whole-grain bread (see page 33), crust removed

Cooking spray

3 tablespoons powdered sugar

1½ teaspoons water

---

1. Preheat the oven to 375°F. Line a baking sheet with parchment paper and set aside.

2. Slice the apple in half, trim the stem, and use a spoon or melon baller to scoop out the seeds. Set aside.

3. In a small bowl, stir together the sugar and cinnamon until well combined. Divide the mixture into two even mounds on the baking sheet at least 6 inches apart. Use a spoon to spread each mound into a circle roughly the size and shape of each apple half.

4. Place the apple halves flesh side down on the cinnamon-sugar mixture. Set aside.

5. Use a rolling pin to roll each slice of bread as flat as possible. Place the bread in the microwave for 20 seconds, until soft and moldable. Lay the slices over each apple and gently mold the bread around the apple.

6. Sprinkle the bread with another pinch of cinnamon and give each slice a mist of cooking spray, which will help keep the bread from drying out. Bake for 20 minutes, until the apples are tender but still have their shape and the sugar has caramelized on the bottom.

7. While the apples bake, stir together the powdered sugar and water. Set aside.

8. When the turnovers are done baking, use a metal spatula to carefully flip them onto a plate so the caramelized sugar is now on top. Allow them to cool slightly, then drizzle each turnover with the frosting. Enjoy warm.

NUTRITION FACTS

FOR 1 SERVING (1 TURNOVER): **CALORIES:** 189 **PROTEIN:** 4g **CARBS:** 38g **FAT:** 1g

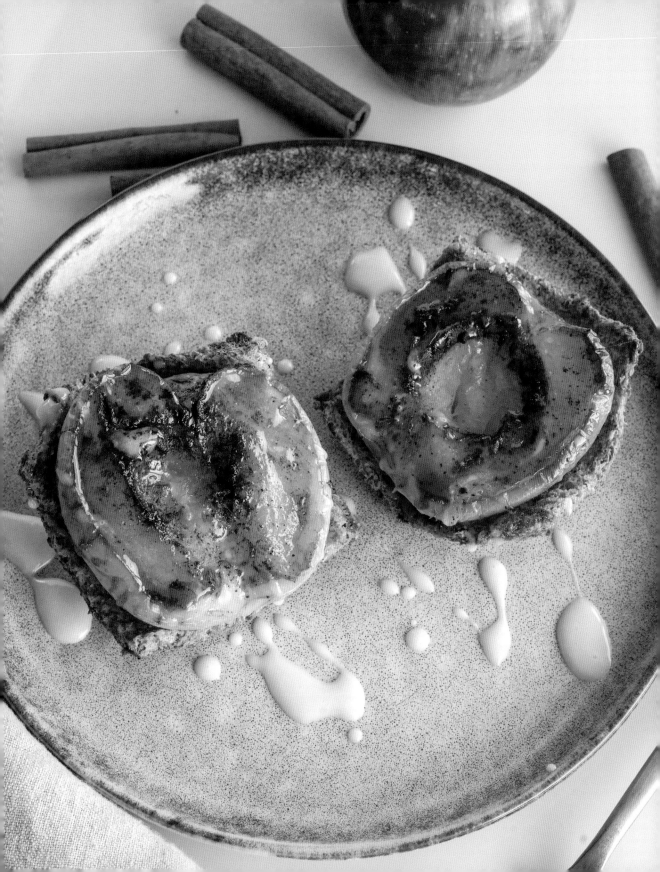

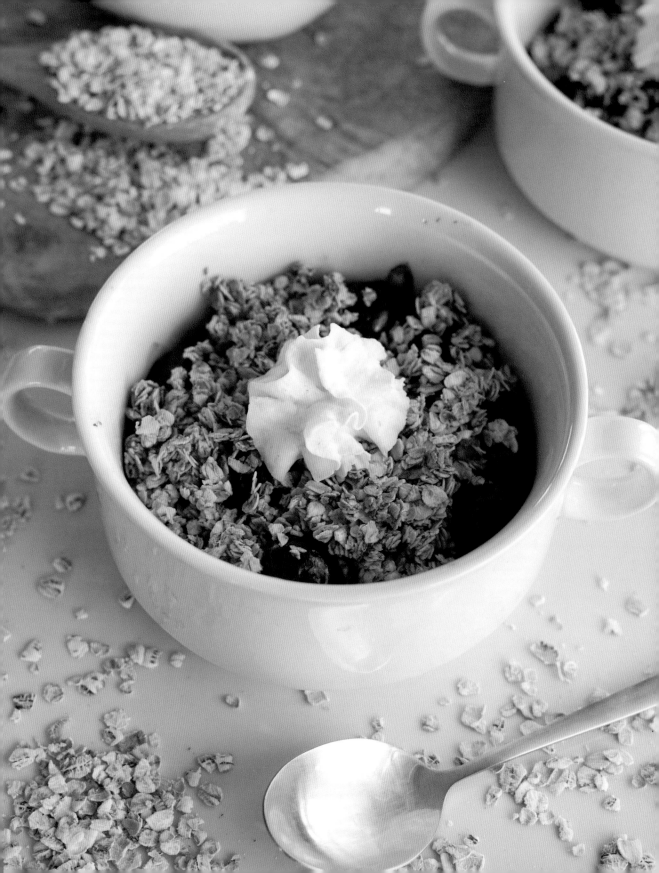

Cherry Pie Bowl

SERVES
1

When I began eating a low-fat, plant-based diet, one of the best discoveries I made was that baked fruit tastes just like the filling of a homemade pie. In this case, I've taken cherries—one of my all-time favorite pie flavors—and topped them with a crisp oat crumble. The vanilla and almond extracts enhance the natural sweetness of the cherries, while the oats give this bowl great crunch. It's easy enough to pull together on a weeknight for a single-serving indulgence, or you can scale this up and serve it as a dessert at summer barbecues.

1 cup fresh cherries, pitted, or
frozen cherries, thawed
¼ cup rolled oats
½ tablespoon maple syrup
¼ teaspoon vanilla extract
¼ teaspoon almond extract
2 tablespoons almond milk whipped
cream (see page 34)

1. Preheat the oven to 400°F.

2. Add the cherries to a small, oven-safe dish and set aside.

3. In a small bowl, combine the oats, maple syrup, vanilla, and almond extract. Mix well to combine.

4. Dollop the oat mixture over the cherries and bake until the oats begin to brown and the cherries are bubbling, about 20 minutes. Allow to cool slightly, then top with the whipped cream and enjoy warm.

NUTRITION FACTS
CALORIES: 210   **PROTEIN:** 4g   **CARBS:** 37g   **FAT:** 2g

Apple Caramel Crisp

SERVES
1

When it comes to quick, easy, intensely satisfying desserts that don't skimp on flavor or substance, it doesn't get much better than fruit baked until hot and bubbly with a crisp oat crust. (It's also why I include variations on this theme, such as the Cherry Pie Bowl on page 241.) When you fold jammy Medjool dates in with the apples to bake, they give this dessert a distinctly caramelesque flavor. Top off the sweet, crunchy oat topping with a mound of whipped cream and you're in business. You could also easily change this recipe up with other fruit, such as blueberries or peaches.

1. Preheat the oven to 400°F.

2. Make the filling: In a small, oven-safe dish, combine the apple, date, maple syrup, lemon juice, vanilla, and apple pie spice.

3. Make the topping: In a small bowl, stir together the oats, maple syrup, vanilla, and cinnamon. Dollop the topping over the prepared filling and bake until the oats begin to brown and the filling is hot and bubbling, 20 minutes.

4. Allow the crisp to cool slightly. Serve warm, topped with the whipped cream.

FOR THE APPLE FILLING

1 small Honeycrisp apple, cored and diced

1 Medjool date, pitted and chopped

1 teaspoon maple syrup

1 teaspoon fresh lemon juice

½ teaspoon vanilla extract

¼ teaspoon apple pie spice

FOR THE OAT TOPPING

¼ cup rolled oats

½ tablespoon maple syrup

½ teaspoon vanilla extract

Pinch of ground cinnamon

2 tablespoons almond milk whipped cream (see page 34)

NUTRITION FACTS
CALORIES: 283   **PROTEIN:** 4g   **CARBS:** 56g   **FAT:** 2g

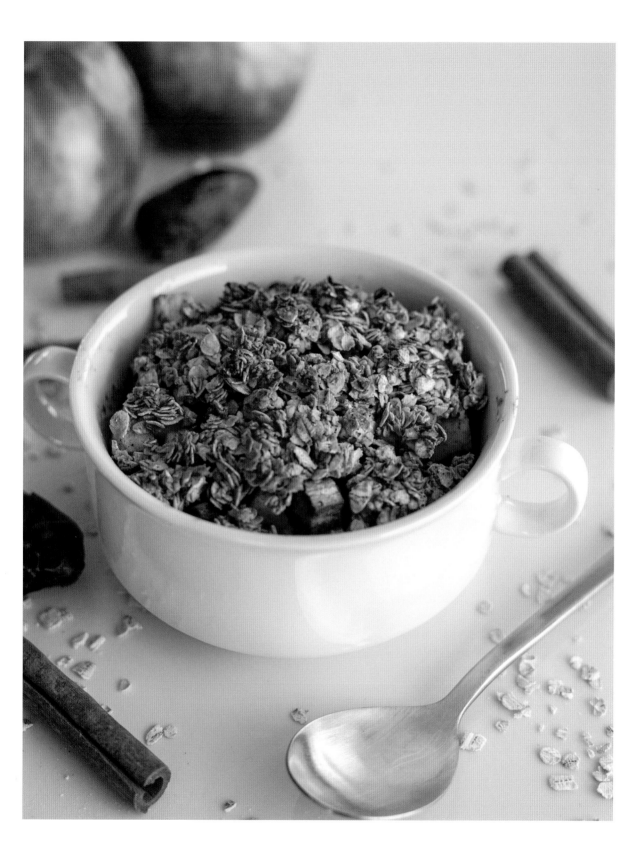

Baked Maple Pecan Pears

SERVES

1

My sister-in-law Amy is a fabulous cook, and one year she made poached pears for Thanksgiving dessert. The first thought I had after seeing them on the table was, There's no way this will be as exciting to eat as apple pie. But, boy, was I wrong! Baking the pears with maple syrup and vanilla deepens their natural flavor and gives them an almost custardy texture. Of course I had to create my own take on Amy's recipe, which calls for popping the pears into the oven instead of babysitting them on the stove. But they're just as deliciously elegant as the original, and would be a great dessert for special occasions.

---

1 Bosc pear
½ tablespoon maple syrup
1 teaspoon fresh lemon juice
½ teaspoon vanilla extract
Pinch of ground cinnamon
1 tablespoon chopped raw pecans

---

1. Preheat the oven to 375°F.

2. Slice the pear in half lengthwise, trim off the stem, and use a small spoon or melon baller to scoop out the seeds. Place the pear halves face-down in a small, oven-safe baking dish.

3. In a small bowl, stir together the maple syrup, lemon juice, and vanilla. Drizzle the syrup mixture over the pears and top with a pinch of cinnamon. Bake until the pears are tender and bubbling, about 10 minutes.

4. While the pears bake, toast the pecans. In a small nonstick pan over medium-high heat, toast the pecans until fragrant, 1 to 2 minutes. Transfer them to a small bowl or plate to cool.

5. When the pears finish baking, transfer them to a plate and sprinkle them with the pecans. Enjoy warm.

NUTRITION FACTS
CALORIES: 180   **PROTEIN:** 1g   **CARBS:** 25g   **FAT:** 5g

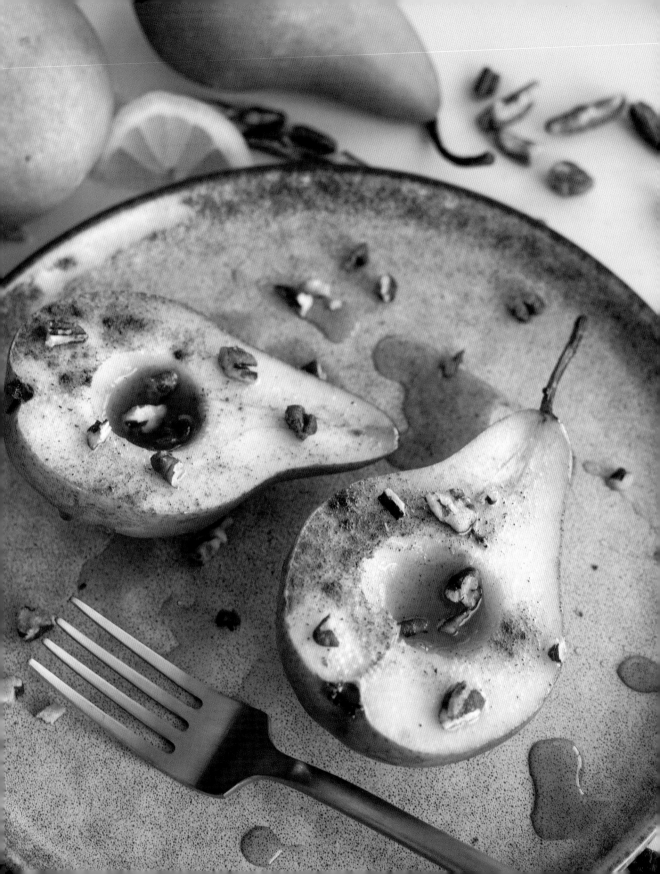

Acknowledgments

I want to thank the incredible people that made this book possible: thank you to my amazing editor, Doris Cooper, for her continual vision and support, to my agent, Janis Donnaud, for her drive and direction, and to my writer, Rachel Holtzman, for her ability to capture my thoughts and intentions in such a clear and beautiful way. Without you or the incredible team at Simon Element, I would not be here.

I would not be here were it not for the profound work of the amazing doctors that helped change my life. All the years I spent struggling with my health and weight were brought to a beautiful end by the tireless dedication of these doctors and their books and teachings. Thank you to Dr. John McDougall; yours was the first book I picked up and the one that started my journey. Thank you, Dr. Neal Barnard, for your incredible work and education on diabetes; you gave me the confidence to change my own prognosis, thus being the first in my family to do so. Thank you to Dr. Joel Fuhrman, Dr. Caldwell Esselstyn, and Dr. T. Colin Campbell; you all have not only positively affected my life, but the lives of thousands of others. Without the work of these incredible doctors, I would be in a much different place than I am today. I am forever grateful.

And a special thank you to Mr. Henry Boyens, who fifteen years ago told me that one day I would write books that would help people. I don't know how you saw into my future way back when I was a young mother struggling with my health and sense of purpose, but your words have stayed with me all these years. Every time I think of you, I smile. The world needs more people like you who are willing to look into others and speak to their potential despite the current circumstances; thank you for seeing something in me at a time when I didn't see it in myself.

Index